Language and Motor Speech Disorders in Adults

HARVEY HALPERN

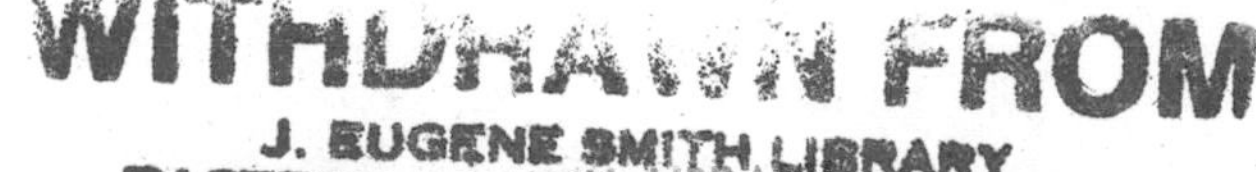

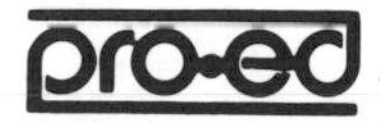

5341 Industrial Oaks Boulevard
Austin, Texas 78735

The PRO-ED studies in communicative disorders

Series editor
HARVEY HALPERN

Library of Congress Cataloging in Publication Data

Halpern, Harvey.
Language and motor speech disorders in adults.

(The PRO-ED studies in communicative disorders)
Bibliography: p.
1. Speech, Disorders of–Diagnosis. 2. Language disorders–Diagnosis.
I. Title. II. Series.
√RC423.H324 1986 616.85'5 86-569
ISBN 089079-089-2

pro-ed
5341 Industrial Oaks Boulevard
Austin, Texas 78735

10 9 8 7 6 5 4 3 2 1 86 87 88 89 90 91

Contents

Preface

The purpose of this monograph is to aid the speech pathologist and others in making a differential diagnosis of speech and language impairment in the adult patient and to provide a framework for speech and language therapy. The material discussed will deal with determining whether a patient has aphasia, generalized intellectual impairment, the language of confusion, the language of schizophrenia, apraxia of speech, dysarthria, or any combination of these disorders. Each of these communication disorders is discussed according to its symptoms, testing procedures, and therapeutic implications.

Language and Motor Speech Disorders in Adults

Introduction

Quite often the speech pathologist is called upon to aid in the differential diagnosis of language and/or speech impairments, to project a prognosis, and then to determine a course of therapy. This evaluation can help decide whether a patient has aphasia, generalized intellectual impairment, confused language, the language of schizophrenia, apraxia of speech, dysarthria, or any combination of these disorders. This information can be very useful, for it helps to determine whether speech therapy is recommended or not and which kind of therapy is applicable. For example, therapy for the aphasic patient involves language training, whereas training for the patient with apraxia of speech might involve a phonetic or motoric approach.

Another advantage is that proper evaluation of the speech and language of a patient can offer the neurologist another diagnostic sign in determining whether a lesion(s) is of focal or diffuse origin. For example, confused language or generalized intellectual impairment is thought to be consistent with diffuse lesions, whereas aphasia and apraxia of speech are generally associated with focal lesions (Mayo Clinic, 1964, pp. 257–258). It is most likely that an attending physician will have made the referral, and information such as onset and type of lesion, accompanying paralysis, visual and hearing problems, and course of medical and other treatment can be gleaned from her.

The factors involved in differentiating among the various groups have been noted (Bayles, Tomoeda, & Caffrey, 1982; Critchley, 1964, 1970, pp. 349–351; Darley, 1964, pp. 36–40; 1982, pp. 8–28, 40; Davis, 1983, pp. 134–147; DiSimoni, Darley, & Aronson, 1977; Halpern, 1978, pp. 379–409; 1980; Halpern, Darley, & Brown, 1973; Halpern & McCartin-Clark, 1984; Holland, 1983, pp. 3–14; Mayo Clinic, 1964, chap. 11, pp. 257–258; Porch, 1971; Stengel, 1964, p. 289; Wertz, 1978, pp. 1–101; 1981; 1984a, pp. 1–77; Wertz, LaPointe, & Rosenbek, 1984, pp. 82–131; and Zangwill, 1964, p. 297).

Aphasia

Aphasia can be defined as a multimodality language disturbance due to brain damage. It is a linguistic deficit that causes the individual to have difficulty in the comprehension and/or formulation of language symbols. This language disturbance is disproportionate to impairment of other neurological, behavioral, and intellectual functions. Aphasia is not generalized intellectual impairment, the language of confusion, the language of schizophrenia, apraxia of speech, or dysarthria, although symptoms of any of these disorders may be similar to aphasia or coexist with it.

Symptoms

Although there is much confusion over the terminology and nomenclature in aphasia, a few definitions seem warranted to start any discussion of aphasic disturbance.

Difficulty in the comprehension of spoken language symbols is generally known as *auditory comprehension deficit*. Here the individual might have greater difficulty in understanding the following: abstract words as opposed to concrete (*justice–jail*); longer words more than shorter (*realistic–real*); infrequently used words as compared with frequent (*domicile–house*); words that sound alike (*fin–thin*); closely associated words (*knife–fork*); and complex sentences that are long, grammatically complex, and include several ideas. There can be a reduced auditory retention span and a general slowness of comprehension.

Alexia is the term used when an individual has an impairment in the comprehension of written symbols (reading). Many of the same disturbances that apply to auditory comprehension deficit can be observed in alexia except that here the difficulty is in comprehension through the visual modality. For example, the individual might confuse words that look alike (*oat–cat*).

Difficulty in the formulation of spoken language symbols can be called *oral expressive aphasia*. This problem is probably influenced by the factors cited under auditory comprehension deficit and manifests itself as the following: a reduced vocabulary with infrequent words mostly gone; telegraphese, usually sparse output with primitive syntax that imparts the message; jargon, unintelligible words that usually follow the phonological rules of the language (*freach*) or intelligible words that bear no relationship to the stimulus; agrammatisms or syntactic errors that involve difficulties with tense, pluralization, prefixes, suffixes, or word order; reduced fluency; excessive fluency; circumlocutions; neologisms, which are made up of new words that are understandable (*skymobile* for *airplane*); semantic paraphasia, which is confusion with closely associated words (saying *knife* for *fork*); phonemic changes or literal paraphasia (*ben* for *pen*); word-finding difficulties; and perseveration, which is the repetition of a response that is no longer appropriate.

An impairment in the formulation of written language symbols is called *agraphia*, and many of the problems and influencing factors cited in the other symptom categories would apply here. For example, if shown a picture of a pen, the patient responds by writing any such closely associated words as *paper*, *ink*, or *pencil*.

Acalculia is a disturbance in handling numerical symbols either through comprehension in listening and/or reading, or formulation in speaking and/or writing.

Types

Aphasia can also be classified into nonfluent aphasia, usually caused by damage to anterior portions of the language-dominant side of the brain, and fluent aphasia, usually caused by damage to posterior portions of the language-dominant side of the brain. Benson (1979, pp. 31–33) and Davis (1983, pp. 19–22), for example, have reviewed both types as follows. Nonfluent aphasia is characterized by (1) decreased output (50 words per minute or less and often fewer than 10 words per minute); (2) increased effort in producing speech; (3) defective articulation (because of the last two characteristics, prosody may be abnormal); (4) decreased phrase length (fewer than 4 words and often only single words); (5) agrammatisms (primitive syntax but a lot of information is conveyed); (6) verbal stereotypy or automatic speech; and (7) awareness of impairment and, as a result, frustration.

Fluent aphasia is characterized by (1) increased output (most are within the normal range of 100–150 words per minute, with some as high as 200 words per minute); (2) effortless production of speech; (3) relatively normal articulation (because of the last two characteristics, prosody may be normal); (4) normal phrase length (about 5 or more words per phrase); (5) apparently normal grammatical structure but a lot of meaningless, empty talk characterized by a lack of substantive words; there are many pauses followed by circumlocutions); (6) many paraphasia of the phonemic or literal, verbal, neologistic, and jargon type; and (7) frequent lack of awareness of the impairment and, as a result, no frustration over the condition.

The nonfluent aphasias would typically include Broca's aphasia, transcortical motor aphasia, global aphasia, and mixed transcortical aphasia or isolation syndrome.

Broca's aphasia is characterized by a sparse output of words and sentences, misarticulations, and agrammatisms. Speech is laborious, filled with many pauses, and telegraphic. Auditory and visual (reading) comprehension is better than speaking, while writing tends to mirror the speaking modality. Repetition of words, phrases, and sentences is poor. Right-sided paralysis is often present, and patients are aware of their difficulties, which can lead to frustration or catastrophic response.

Transcortical motor aphasia is similar to Broca's aphasia with the exception that these patients have the ability to repeat words, phrases, and sentences. It is a relatively rare syndrome.

Global aphasia consists of a severe impairment in auditory comprehension, reading, speaking, and writing. Patients try to communicate but often can produce only verbal stereotypes and automatic speech. Repetition of words, phrases, and sentences is defective.

Mixed transcortical aphasia or isolation syndrome is similar to global aphasia except that these patients can repeat and show echolalia of words, phrases, and sentences. It is a relatively rare syndrome (Benson, 1979, pp. 90–92).

The fluent aphasias would typically include Wernicke's aphasia, transcortical sensory aphasia, conduction aphasia, and anomic aphasia.

Wernicke's aphasia is characterized by fluent paraphasia and generally well-articulated speech. Jargon, neologisms, and empty speech are common features. Auditory and visual (reading) comprehension as well as writing are impaired. Repetition of words, phrases, and sentences is poor. Patients show little or no other neurologic signs and are often unaware of their errors, which leads to little frustration. On the other hand, some of these patients can become suspicious or even paranoid about their circumstances.

Transcortical sensory aphasia is similar to Wernicke's aphasia except that these patients have the ability to repeat and show echolalia of words, phrases, and sentences. It is a relatively rare syndrome.

Conduction aphasia consists of fluent verbal and phonemic paraphasic speech, although usually less severe than that of the Wernicke's aphasic. Auditory and visual (reading) comprehension is relatively good while writing is defective. Repetition of words, phrases, and sentences is disproportionately severely impaired in relation to the level of fluency in spontaneous speech and the near normal level of auditory comprehension. Other motor signs may be present, and because of the patient's awareness of errors, his speech can be filled with unsuccessful attempts at self-correction.

Anomic aphasia is characterized by fluent, well-articulated, mildly paraphasic, grammatically intact, and somewhat empty speech. The outstanding symptom is a naming or word-finding problem that can affect any of the modalities. Generally, if other symptoms appear, they do so mildly in the various modalities. These patients have no difficulty with repetition of words, phrases, and sentences. They know when they are in error, and because of unsuccessful attempts at self-correction, they often become frustrated.

For a further review of the various symptoms and classifications of aphasia, the reader is referred to Benson (1979, pp. 65–106), Berndt and Caramazza (1981, pp. 157–182), Blumstein (1981, pp. 129–155), Buckingham (1981, pp. 188–214), Caramazza (1984), Collins (1983), Damasio (1981, pp. 51–65), Davis (1983, pp. 20–22), Eisenson (1984, pp. 1–36, 103–116), Fitch-West (1984, pp. 384–396), Goodglass and Kaplan (1983), Helm-Estabrooks (1984, pp. 159–176), Holland (1982b, pp. 434–438), Horner (1984, pp. 133–157), Kertesz (1979), Lesser (1978), Linebaugh (1984a, pp. 113–131), Riedel (1981, pp. 215–269), and Schwartz (1984).

Etiology

As was stated in the definition, aphasia is caused by brain damage most likely of focal origin. A major cause of aphasia in middle and old age is the cerebrovascular accident. Cerebrovascular accidents consist of thromboses, embolisms, aneurysms, hemorrhages, and ischemias. A cerebral thrombosis is an occlusion of an artery to the brain by a clot. A cerebral embolus is a clot formed elsewhere and finally lodging in the brain. An aneurysm is a swelling or ballooning of a cranial artery. A cerebral hemorrhage is the rupture of a blood vessel with subsequent bleeding into the brain. Ischemia refers to deficient circulation in the brain. All of the cerebrovascular accidents have one thing in common: they deprive the brain of oxygen and circulation, thus causing brain damage.

Trauma to the brain is another major cause of aphasia. Gunshot wounds, automobile accidents, and falls are most likely involved in physical trauma to the brain. Brain tumors, both malignant and nonmalignant, are associated with causing aphasia. Quite often the extirpation of a brain tumor will cause aphasia. Abscesses, infectious diseases, and degenerative diseases of the brain can also result in aphasia. Reviews of etiology of aphasia can be found in Benson (1979, pp. 18–29), Davis (1983, pp. 26–40), Eisenson (1984, pp. 37–71), Levin (1981, pp. 427–463), and Stein (1981, pp. 15–29).

Diagnosis

Keeping in mind the previously mentioned factors, it is quite possible to differentiate the language and motor speech disorders in adults by using the evaluative instruments employed with aphasia. In a book edited by Darley (1979), an evaluation is made of a number of tests used in aphasia. They include the following: Aphasia Language Performance Scales (ALPS) (Keenan & Brassell, 1975); Boston Diagnostic Aphasia Examination (BDAE) (Goodglass & Kaplan, 1983); Examining for Aphasia (Eisenson, 1954); the Functional Communication Profile (FCP) (Sarno, 1969); the Language Modalities Test for Aphasia (LMTA) (Wepman & Jones, 1961); the Minnesota Test for Differential Diagnosis of Aphasia (MTDDA) (Schuell, 1972); Neurosensory Center Comprehensive Examination for Aphasia (NCCEA) (Spreen & Benton, 1969); Porch Index of Communicative Ability (PICA) (Porch, 1971); Sklar Aphasia Scale (SAS) (Sklar, 1966); the Token Test (DeRenzi & Vignolo, 1962); and the Word Fluency Measure (Borkowsky, Benton, & Spreen, 1967).

Added to that list but not evaluated in the Darley (1979) book are the following: Auditory Comprehension Test for Sentences (ACTS) (Shewan, 1980); Communicative Abilities in Daily Living (CADL) (Holland, 1980); Multilingual Aphasia Examination (MAE) (Benton & Hamsher, 1978); Reading Comprehension Battery for Aphasia (RCBA) (LaPointe & Horner, 1980); the Reporter's Test (DeRenzi & Ferrari, 1978); and the Western Aphasia Battery (WAB) (Kertesz & Poole, 1974). Scoring procedures and diagnostic nomenclature will vary depending upon the test that is used for evaluation.

Test items related to discovering the symptoms of a generalized intellectual impairment, the language of confusion, the language of schizophrenia, apraxia of speech, and dysarthria are discussed later in this paper. Those items can be added to any of the aphasia tests mentioned above in order to make a differential diagnosis.

Most of the tests used in aphasia evaluate all four modalities. Each modality is tested individually, with stimulus items generally ranging from simple to more complex. For example, auditory comprehension might be tested by the examiner saying single words, multiple words, sentences, and paragraphs to the patient (e.g, "Point to the window"). The patient would respond through pointing, nodding, or gesturing to the auditory stimuli. Visual comprehension (reading) is tested by presenting printed material in the form of words, sentences, and paragraphs (e.g., "Do cows fly?") to the patient and having her respond by pointing, nodding, gesturing, circling, or underlining. Oral expression is tested by having the patient produce serial speech (reciting the alphabet, days of the week, etc.), name pictures or objects, repeat words after the examiner, define words and sentences, and talk spontaneously about everyday activities. Writing is tested by having the patient write words to dictation, write down the name of an object or an item shown in a picture, and write a narrative from an action picture. Tests that evaluate the four modalities generally in the manner described would include the ALPS, BDAE, Examining for Aphasia, LMTA, MTDDA, MEA, NCCEA, PICA, SAS, and the WAB.

Some tests evaluate functional language through the four modalities. Many times these tests are used as an adjunct to the more traditional ones used in aphasia and would include the CADL and the FCP. Test items elicit language related to everyday activities (greetings, shopping, etc.), and these tests are administered in a relatively informal manner. The authors of those tests feel that because of the emphasis on functional language and the informal setting, the psychological barriers of tension and anxiety that accompany formal test-taking would be ameliorated.

Other tests evaluate the patient's language abilities only through one modality. Usually these tests evaluate in an in-depth manner and are quite sensitive, thus enabling the detection of even the mildest language impairment. These tests are mostly used as adjuncts to the more traditional ones and include ACTS (auditory), RCBA (reading), the Reporters Test (oral expression), the Token Test (auditory), and the Word Fluency Measure (oral expression).

Reviews of testing procedures in aphasia can be found in Chapey (1981a, pp. 31–84), Darley (1982, pp. 55–85), Davis (1983, pp. 127–208), Fitch-West (1984, pp. 403–410), Ludlow (1983, pp. 75–81), Spreen and Risser (1981, pp. 67–128), Tikofsky (1984, pp. 117–149), and Wertz (1978, pp. 1–101; 1981; 1984a, pp. 1–77).

With a view toward diagnosis, Halpern, Darley, and Brown (1973) examined four groups of patients, each group demonstrating a different neurogenic disorder of communication, for impairment in 10 intellectual and language categories. The four groups were aphasia, generalized intellectual impairment, the language of confusion, and apraxia of speech. Each had been given a standard neurologic examination and a language examination that was an adaptation of Schuell's (1957) short examination of aphasia.

The 10 language and intellectual categories were as follows: auditory retention span; auditory comprehension; reading comprehension; naming; writing words to dictation; arithmetic; syntax (errors included use of improper grammatical inflection, such as tense or number, and addition or deletion of or substitution for syntactic words); adequacy (erroneous responses included substitution, deletion, and addition of substantive words; the degree of elaboration of the response also entered into the judgment of adequacy); relevance (errors were bizarre responses that appeared unrelated to the stimulus; patient unaware of error and makes no attempt to self-correct); and fluency (errors included excessive hesitation and sparseness in responses).

Analysis of the speech and language data indicated that the group with aphasia was differentiated from the others by impairment of auditory retention span and a lack of fluency. The neurological data showed that the aphasia was of variable onset and duration and was associated in 9 cases with infarcts or tumors in predominantly posterior lesions. (In this study, 7 patients had a rapid onset, less than 10 days, and 3 patients had a slow onset. This is typical, since onset of aphasia is usually rapid.)

Using the same language examination, Halpern and McCartin-Clark (1984) tested 61 aphasic and 61 schizophrenic subjects. They found that the language categories of strongest differentiating value were writing words to dictation, naming, syntax (where aphasic subjects were more impaired in all three) and relevance (where schizophrenic subjects were more impaired, especially on the less structured or more open-ended portions, such as defining words and proverbs, explaining three things that every good citizen should do, responding to an action picture, or elaborating a typical day). To a lesser extent, other differentiating language features were auditory retention span, overall language ability (where aphasic subjects were more impaired in both), and fluency (where aphasic subjects were more nonfluent).

Prognosis

Before deciding on who would make a good candidate for therapy or providing information to patients and their families about the prospects for improvement, there are a number of prognostic indicators that might give some insight into these processes. These indicators might also predict improvement through spontaneous recovery.

Although the prognostic factors cited are gleaned from the literature in aphasia, many of these indicators might be applicable to patients with the other communication disorders.

The prognostic indicators have been outlined by Brookshire (1983), Darley (1972; 1982, pp. 127–143), Davis (1983, pp. 220–237), Eisenson (1949; 1981, pp. 85–101; 1984, pp. 150–166), Emerick and Hatten (1974, pp. 249–251), Fitch-West (1984, pp. 396–403), Marshall and Phillips (1983), J. Sarno (1981, pp. 465–484), M. Sarno (1981, pp. 485–529), Vignolo (1964), Wepman (1953), Wertz (1983a, pp. 196–220), and Wertz, LaPointe, and Rosenbek (1984, pp. 138–142). They consist of the following:

1. The younger the patient, the better the prognosis.
2. The sooner the patient enters therapy from the time of onset of aphasia, the better the prognosis.
3. The less extensive the neurological damage, the better the prognosis.

4. Trauma as a cause of aphasia seems to warrant a better prognosis than the cerebrovascular accidents.
5. If the aphasic patient has the will to improve and accept his limitations, the prognosis is better.
6. If the family of the aphasic patient has the proper attitude and provides encouragement to the patient, the prognosis is better.
7. The milder the language impairment at the initial evaluation, the better the prognosis.
8. If the patient receives a longer and more intense period of speech and language therapy, the prognosis is better.
9. The better the physical condition with no sensory defects, the better the prognosis.

Darley (1982, pp. 102–103) has cited several studies indicating that when dysarthria accompanies aphasia, the prognosis is poorer. However, these studies were not in agreement about prognosis when apraxia of speech accompanies aphasia. Although there are always exceptions, these prognostic factors might provide insight and guidelines for therapy and help in guidance and counselling procedures with the family. If the speech pathologist is in doubt about whether to recommend therapy, my suggestion would be to recommend it. A patient can always be released from therapy if it does not prove to be beneficial, and nothing is really lost. Finally, if a complete evaluation is not made during the initial diagnostic session, but it is enough for a limited diagnosis, I would recommend therapy for the patient. This would provide time for an ongoing and complete diagnosis in addition to the benefits of therapy.

The literature has been reviewed by Darley (1972; 1982, chap. 4), Eisenson (1984, pp. 160–162), Fitch-West (1984, pp. 431–437), Hilton and Kraetschmer (1983), LaPointe (1978, pp. 129–190), M. Sarno (1981, chap. 17), and Wertz (1983a, pp. 196–220). Basso, Capitani, and Vignolo (1979) and Wertz et al. (1981) have investigated variables on the efficacy of aphasia therapy. Although the final word is not in, it seems that speech and language therapy of the aphasic patient is beneficial for language recovery.

Therapy

Approaches to aphasia therapy have generally been divided into two schools of thought: the stimulation method and the programmed instruction method. Darley (1972; 1982, pp. 186–278) and M. Sarno (1981, chap. 17) review both methods. As Darley (1972) has stated, "In the stimulation approach the goal of therapy is to stimulate the patient to produce cortical integrations necessary for language, not to educate or reeducate him and not to convey specific new learning or new vocabulary. . . . That stimulus must be adequate and it must get into the brain.

It involves repetitive sensory stimulation, each stimulus eliciting a response" (pp. 12–13). For specifics and a further elaboration of this method of aphasia therapy, the reader is referred to Chapey (1981b, pp. 155–167; 1983). Darley (1982, chaps. 5–6), Davis and Wilcox (1981), Duffy (1981), LaPointe (1978), Lubinski (1981), Martin (1981), Muma and McNeil (1981), Mysak and Guarino (1981), Schuell, Jenkins, and Jimenez-Pabon (1964), and Wepman (1951).

Duffy (1981, pp. 105–139) has reviewed and analyzed the stimulation approaches to aphasia therapy. He notes that the use of intensive controlled auditory stimulation is supported by the following: (1) sensory stimulation affects brain activities; (2) repeated sensory stimuli are essential for the organization, storage, and retrieval of language patterns in the brain; (3) the auditory system is of prime importance for language acquisition and for processing information and feedback in ongoing functional language; (4) nearly all aphasic patients have auditory deficits, and recovery in this modality will help the other modalities; (5) because of its crucial link to language, gains made through the auditory modality will extend to all other input and output language channels.

Duffy (1981, pp. 105–139) further reviews the general principles of the stimulation method. They are as follows: (1) intensive auditory stimulation should be used along with the other modalities; (2) the stimulus must be adequate and get into the brain; (3) repetitive sensory stimulation should be used; (4) each stimulus should elicit a response; (5) responses should be elicited and not forced; (6) a maximum number of responses should be elicited; a large number of adequate responses indicates a large number of adequate stimuli; (7) feedback about accuracy of response should be provided when such feedback appears beneficial; (8) work should proceed systematically and intensively; (9) sessions should begin with relatively easy, familiar tasks and proceed to more difficult tasks after the patient experiences success; (10) the examiner should use abundant and varied materials and present them in the proper manner; (11) new materials and procedures should be extensions of familiar materials and procedures.

The structure of stimulation listed below follows Duffy's (1981, pp. 112–130) outline. Much of the research surrounding each factor can be found in Darley (1982, pp. 186–236), Duffy (1981, pp. 112–130), and Fitch-West (1984, pp. 411–424).

1. Auditory perceptual clarity (volume and noise). Reducing noise or working in quiet facilitates language performance. Increasing volume is not useful except in specific cases.

2. Nonlinguistic visual-perceptual clarity (dimensionality, size, color, content, ambiguity, operativity). Be clear, realistic, and redundant. The most potent

visual stimuli appear to be characterized by three-dimensionality, color, lack of ambiguity, operativity, and redundant physical properties.

3. Linguistic visual-perceptual clarity (size and form). Large print seems better; be aware of idiosyncratic preference.
4. Method of delivery of auditory stimulation. Auditory stimulation that is direct, binaural, and free-field is best.
5. Discriminability (semantic, auditory, visual). The best approach is to select stimuli that offer few response alternatives.
6. Stimulus repetition. Repetition of stimuli after the incorrect response appears to increase adequate responses.
7. Rate and pause. Speak slowly with a slow overall rate. Pause at appropriate intervals to help auditory retention and reduce rate of phoneme production by prolonging words.
8. Length (a factor in all modalities). Through the visual modality, short words, sentences, and paragraphs are better; through the auditory modality, shorter phrases, sentences, and paragraphs are better. Length may not be a factor at the word level. Redundancy can overcome the limitations of length.
9. Combined sensory modalities. The best is combined auditory and visual stimulation. This helps the single modalities and is a good starting point. Using the tactile modality also helps. The multimodality stimulus provides redundancy and additional cues for the patient. Don't overload with too much multimodality stimulation. It can cause distraction and exceed the capacity of the patient. Beukelman, Yorkston, and Waugh (1980) have found that aphasic patients are more successful when given combined verbal and pantomimed instructions than when given these instructions individually.
10. Cues, prompts, and prestimulation. This is highly dependent on the patient.
11. Frequency and meaningfulness. The more meaningful (natural communicative context or functional) the stimuli, the greater the chance of a correct response.
12. Abstractness. A possible factor, but one overcome by frequency, redundancy, and operativity.
13. Part of speech. Verbs, adjectives, adverbs, and nouns may be easier (if frequency is controlled) than conjunctions, articles, and prepositions. Semantic word categories (naming of objects, colors, letters, action numbers) are debatable.

14. Grammatical considerations. There is a hierarchy of grammatical difficulty that affects all the aphasias.

15. Stress. This factor appears tied to saliency, word order, and grammatical complexity.

16. Order of difficulty. Begin with familiar, easy tasks, then proceed to less familiar and more difficult ones, and end with tasks that result in a great deal of success.

17. Psychological and physical factors. Patients do better when not suffering from tension or fatigue. Tompkins, Marshall, and Phillips (1980) found that mornings are better than afternoons for scheduling therapy.

18. Pattern of auditory deficit. According to Brookshire (1978, pp. 103–128), patients can show any of the following: slow rise time (miss initial portions); noise build-up (miss final portions); retention deficit (length causes problems); information capacity deficit (too many ideas in sentences); intermittent auditory imperception (fades in and out randomly).

Concerning response characteristics, short responses are easier for the patient. The speech pathologist should choose the modality easiest for the patient and see whether the patient responds best in unison with the stimulus, immediately following a stimulus, or after a delay. The response characteristics of accuracy, recognition, and attempts at correction should all be considered. Marshall and Tompkins (1981) offer a good review of the self-cueing and self-correction behaviors of aphasic patients. The therapist can give patients feedback on their responses by letting them know how they are doing.

Darley (1972) and M. Sarno (1981, chap. 17) further noted that the programmed instruction method, on the contrary, views language rehabilitation as an educative process and applies, in a rigorous way, operant conditioning methods drawn from psycholinguistic analysis to guide the content and order of presentation of the linguistic elements taught. It is based on the belief that there are several distinguishable stages of learning, including recognition, imitation, repetition of the model based on memory of the echoed performance, and, finally, spontaneous selection of response from a repertoire of learned responses. For specifics and a further elaboration of this method of aphasia therapy, the reader is referred to the work done by Brookshire (1967), Costello (1977), DiCarlo (1980), Fitch and Cross (1983), Goldfarb (1981), Holland (1970), and Seron, DeLoche, Moulard, and Rouselle (1980).

In a rather exciting combination of the two approaches, LaPointe (1977) proposes the Base-Ten Programmed Stimulation Method. Included in this method are the programmed operant features of clearly defined tasks, baseline performance measurement, and session-by-session progress-plotting of the aphasia patient. This is combined with the many features of the stimulation method designed to elicit many responses from aphasic patients. With the programmed stimulation approach, speech and language tasks are composed of 10 stimulus items, which are scored and plotted during 10 therapy sessions. LaPointe also presents a discussion of the compensatory-facilitative and self-cueing strategies useful for some aphasic patients in verbal production and auditory comprehension.

Darley (1982, chaps. 5–6), Duffy (1981), Eisenson (1984, pp. 179–206), Fitch-West (1984, pp. 378–445), LaPointe (1978, pp. 129–190), M. Sarno (1981, chap. 17), and Wertz (1978, 1981) review some of the considerations in focusing aphasia therapy. They discuss the stimuli, stimulus modes, response modes, temporal relation of stimulus and response, facilitators, and methods in aphasia therapy. Brookshire (1978) and Marshall (1981) offer some concepts of aphasia therapy with auditory comprehension problems. Sparks (1981) and Sparks and Holland (1976) have reported success in using melodic intonation therapy with mildly to moderately impaired aphasic patients. The intoned pattern is based on one of several speech prosody patterns that are reasonably obvious for a given sentence, depending on the inference intended. The three elements are the melodic line, the rhythm, and the points of stress. Davis and Wilcox (1981) propose a method of therapy called Promoting Aphasics' Communicative Effectiveness (PACE), which incorporates components of face-to-face conversation and is based upon pragmatic language (language used in context). Rollin (1984, pp. 252–282) describes a plan of family therapy for the aphasic adult.

Porch (1981) offers a plan for aphasia therapy based on PICA test results. DiSimoni (1981) proposes alternative or augmentative systems to communication such as communication boards, sign language (Guilford, Scheuerle, & Shirek, 1982), and mechanical communication devices. Aten, Caliguiri, and Holland (1982) and Holland (1982a) suggest using functional communication in aphasia group therapy. Darley (1982, chap. 6) and M. Sarno (1981, chap. 17) review specific techniques geared for the global aphasic. One such method is visual action therapy (Helm & Benson, 1978; Helm-Estabrooks, Fitzpatrick, & Barresi, 1982), whereby the patient is taught to associate ideographic forms with specific objects (cup, razor, etc.) and actions. Another method is visual communication therapy (Gardner, Zurif, Berry, & Baker, 1976), which is designed to teach the global aphasic artificial language using a system of arbitrary symbols representing syntactic and lexical components. The Helm Elicited Language Program for Syntax Stimulation (Estabrooks, 1981) is an approach designed to stimulate the agrammatic or paragrammatic aphasics' access to syntactical knowledge. Darley (1982, chap. 6) further surveys group therapy procedures that involve socializing experiences, listening to lectures, holding discussions, going on excursions, working puzzles, group singing, participating in word lotto and proverb games, manipulating puppets, preparing tape recordings using functional conversation, focusing on adjustment problems, and utilizing daily psychotherapy.

Success in group therapy for aphasic patients has recently been reported by Aten, Caligiuri, and Holland (1982), Eisenson (1984, pp. 232–239), Fitch-West (1984, pp. 428–431), and Wertz et al. (1981).

Taylor (1964) has reviewed the nonspecific stimulation or the spontaneous recovery approach, which involves no approach at all. These nonspecific stimulation approaches would include the following: (1) the environment stimulation approach, in which everybody around the patient talks as much as possible; (2) the rapport approach, in which a warm relationship is established between the clinician and the patient without regard to the content or method of presentation of stimuli; (3) the socialization approach or coffee-hour treatment, in which group sessions include singing, crafts, hobbies, games, telling jokes, and playing pranks; (4) the psychotherapeutic approach, whereby group work is focused on problems such as anxiety and loss of self-esteem, with little direct attempt to retain language; and (5) the interest approach, in which patients are motivated by materials relating to their previous interests and activities. These nonspecific stimulation approaches have been used rather widely in the past. At present, they are probably used as adjuncts to the current forms of aphasia therapy. Additional reviews of aphasia therapy can be found in Davis (1983, pp. 238–289), Eisenson (1984, pp. 207–231), Fitch-West (1984, pp. 378–445), Helm-Estabrooks (1983, pp. 229–238), Hilton and Kraetschmer (1983), Hoops (1980, pp. 337–375), LaPointe (1978, pp. 129–190; 1983, pp. 127–136), Rosenbek (1983, pp. 317–325), and Wertz (1981; 1983a, pp. 196–220; 1983b).

Summing up, aphasia is a linguistic disturbance that affects the person's receptive and expressive language ability. Language is affected through the modalities unevenly; that is, some are better than others. Except for the patient with a severe auditory comprehension deficit, who can show little or no awareness of the problem, most aphasic patients want to communicate and become frustrated when they cannot. Semantic and syntactic errors are quite typical of aphasic responses, and, although language structure is off, thought and content are relevant to the situation. The patient's answers are not bizarre.

Generalized Intellectual Impairment

A generalized intellectual impairment (GII) implies a general lowering of intellectual functions. Performance on language tasks and other mental tasks are approximately equally defective. The patient usually exhibits an across-the-board depression of mental faculties, personality changes, emotional lability, dull and bland behavior, and memory loss (Darley, 1964, p. 39; Halpern, Darley, & Brown, 1973; Mayo Clinic, 1964, pp. 238–239; Wertz, 1978, pp. 1–101; 1984a, pp. 1–77). GII in its early stages can resemble normal behavior or sometimes a mild aphasia.

Symptoms

According to Wertz (1978, pp. 1–101; 1984a, pp. 1–77), the speech pathologist diagnoses the language of GII, and the neurologist and psychologist diagnose dementia. Cortical dementia is identified by problems in language, cognition, visuospatial (motor) abilities, and behavior. Language problems include a restricted vocabulary that is limited to small talk and stereotyped clichés. Perseveration (Gewirth, Shindler, & Hier, 1984), word-finding difficulty, semantic errors, and naming problems are also present. Deficits in cognition (Davis, 1983, p. 136) usually involve memory loss, time and place disorientation, intellectual decline, and faulty judgment. The patient's personality behavior can be dull and bland and can also show emotional lability at times. Kaszniak, Garron, and Fox (1979) and Wilson, Kaszniak, and Fox (1981) found that recent memory and remote memory can be affected in the dementia patient. Recently, Bentin, Silverberg, and Gordon (1981) found that dementia patients showed greater deficits in right-hemisphere functioning (spatial orientation and direction, facial recall, patterns, pictures or scenes, and in grasping new global concepts) than in left-hemisphere functioning (logical thought, serial or temporal processing, and verbal abilities). An additional review of cortical dementia can be found in Cummings and Benson (1983, pp. 35–72).

Types

Bayles, Tomoeda, and Caffrey (1982) and Obler and Albert (1981, pp. 385–398) have delineated three stages in cortical dementia. During the mild stage, the patient senses a decline, becomes apologetic, and is reluctant to be tested. Frequently he is disoriented to time, and his memory for recent events has begun to fail. The patient relies heavily on overlearned situations and stereotypical utterances and is often unable to generate sequences of related ideas. In this stage, the patient might resemble the Wernicke's patient; however, the Wernicke's patient cannot repeat whereas the dementia patient often can.

Bayles, Tomoeda, and Caffrey (1982) point out that the dementia patient, in this stage, begins to exhibit impairment semantically (slightly reduced vocabulary; word-finding difficulties; increased use of automatisms and clichés) and pragmatically (mild loss of desire to communicate; occasional disinhibitions), whereas syntactically and phonologically he is intact.

During the moderate stage, the patient has a more noticeable memory and orientation to time and place impairment. The patient is more perseverative, nonmeaningful, and does not correct his own errors. Bayles, Tomoeda, and Caffrey (1982) have noted that the dementia patient, in this stage, shows further impairment semantically (significantly reduced vocabulary; naming errors usually semantically and visually related; verbal paraphasias evident in discourse), shows some impairment syntactically (reduction in syntactic complexity and completeness), shows further impairment pragmatically (declining sensitivity to context; diminished eye contact; egocentricity), whereas phonologically he is generally intact.

Because of difficulty with abstraction, utterances are usually concrete. Repetition begins to break down, and the patient shows circumlocutions and anomic difficulties. Eye contact begins to diminish, and there is lots of touching of objects, indicating that the pragmatics of communication are inappropriate. Wilson et al. (1982) found that dementia patients show a deficit in the retention of facial information. The aphasic patient would probably be adequate in this area.

In the advanced stage, patients are very much disoriented to time, place, and person, and fail to recognize family and friends. They are unable to carry out the routines of life and require extensive personal care. Many times they will make spontaneous corrections of syntactic and phonologic errors but without awareness. They have brief moments when stimuli appear to be comprehended, but for the most part they will neither comprehend nor self-correct any errors. Their phonology is generally correct; syntax may be disturbed, but not as disturbed as the semantic aspects of language (Bayles, 1982; Bayles & Boone, 1982). It seems that the phonologic and syntactic aspects remain relatively unimpaired while the semantic and pragmatic aspects of language are very much impaired. The referential aspects of language are very disturbed while the mechanics of speech production are not disturbed unless a subcortical degeneration process has taken place. In some cases, the patient could be mute except for jargon.

Bayles, Tomoeda, and Caffrey (1982) point out that the dementia patient, in this stage, shows further impairment semantically (markedly reduced vocabulary; frequent unrelated misnamings; jargon common), further impairment syntactically (many inappropriate word combinations), further impairment pragmatically (nonadherence to conventional rules; poor eye contact; lack of social awareness; inability to form a purposeful intention), and some impairment phonologically (occasional phonemic paraphasias and neologisms; sometimes jargon). Additional reviews of the speech and language in dementia can be found in Bayles (1984, pp. 209–244), Cummings and Benson (1983, pp. 40–43), and Obler and Albert (1981, pp. 385–398).

Etiology

The etiology of cortical dementia is brain damage that is diffuse, degenerative, and progressive as typified by Alzheimer's disease, which makes up the highest incidence (50%) of all dementia cases. Multiinfarct dementia, which is vascular in origin, is the second highest in incidence and accounts for between 14% and 20% of dementia cases. Another 16% to 20% of dementia patients suffer from both Alzheimer's and multiinfarct diseases. The cause of Alzheimer's disease is unknown, but some nonmutually exclusive factors such as accumulation of environmental toxins, heredity, virus, and old age have been suggested (Bayles, Tomoeda, & Caffrey, 1982).

Subcortical dementia is characterized by a gradual decline in cognitive abilities without any appreciable loss in associational cortical areas (language). The patient has emotional and personality changes, which are typically inertia or apathy. Memory disorders are present, and the patient has a defective ability to manipulate acquired knowledge. There is also a general slowness of information-processing through the visual or auditory modality. The speech disturbance is usually dysarthric while language tends toward the concrete. The etiology of subcortical dementia is brain damage that is diffuse, degenerative, and progressive. Parkinson's disease and Huntington's disease are typical causes of this dementia. Cummings and Benson (1983, pp. 35–273) offer a comprehensive review of the etiologies associated with cortical and subcortical dementia.

Diagnosis

In testing for generalized intellectual impairment, questions relating to time and place orientation and simple general information can be used along with the tests used in aphasia evaluation. Where necessary, the different modalities should be used for eliciting an answer. Even when the clinician uses the different modalities, the patient will miss many easy questions such as: What day is it? What month? What is today's date? What year? Where are you now? What city? What state? Why are you here? In addition to these orientation questions, the clinician can ask general information questions such as: When do we celebrate Christmas? What is the capital of the United States? Who is the president of the United States? Before him? Who discovered America? When? How many states are there in the United States? Who was the first president of the United States? Who was president during the Civil War? Who invented Mickey Mouse and Donald Duck? What country is immediately north of the United States? Who was Helen Keller?

Critchley (1970, pp. 349–351) has stated that in cases of dementia language impairment essentially entails a poverty of language due to inaccessibility of the speaking, writing, and reading vocabulary. With advancing mental inelasticity and memory loss, words utilized by dementia patients become severely restricted in conversation and, to a somewhat lesser extent, in writing. The difficulty in word-finding differs from the anomia of aphasic patients. The dementia patient does not necessarily show hesitancy in naming objects. Semantic errors in naming do not occur nor do neologisms and substitutions. On the other hand, dementia patients find it difficult to name, unless the real object is before them. They lapse into a sort of concrete attitude.

Critchley further noted that "a patient with early dementia (GII) may preserve a facade of normalcy for quite a long time, by resorting to small talk. As time goes by, his repertoire of things to say becomes more limited and more stereotyped . . . 'more laced with clichés and set phrases.' Later the subject remains taciturn unless directly addressed. This social seclusion does not embarrass or perturb the patient" (p. 350). Perserveration, which might be indicative of an ideational rigidity, is also present in written and spoken language.

Stengel (1964) and Zangwill (1964) have also indicated that in a question-and-answer session the GII patient may be able to answer simple, ordinary, concrete questions, but not those of a more abstract nature. Typically he is not distressed and exhibits dull and bland behavior toward the situation.

Appell, Kertesz, and Fisman (1982) found that the Alzheimer's patients showed symptoms that resembled those of Wernicke's aphasia and transcortical sensory aphasia more than they resembled those of Broca's aphasia or transcortical motor aphasia. Obler, Albert, Estabrooks, and Nicholas (1982) point out that more neologisms and verbal paraphasia exist in Wernicke's aphasia, while the Alzheimer's patient shows more logical conjunctions and comments.

Benson (1979, p. 160) states that anomia in aphasic patients separates them from dementia patients. Horner et al. (1982) and Obler and Albert (1981, p. 391) have noted that the naming errors of the dementia patient are more likely due to visual misperceptions than the naming errors of aphasic patients, which are mostly of a semantic or phonological nature. Bayles and Tomoeda (1983) and Martin and Fedio (1983) have also noted a naming problem in dementia, which gets worse as the disease progresses.

Bayles, Tomoeda, and Caffrey (1982) have noted that the dementia patient in the mild stage exhibits some semantic and pragmatic impairment; in the moderate stage, further semantic and pragmatic impairment and some syntactic impairment; and in the advanced stage, further semantic, pragmatic, and syntactic impairment and some phonologic impairment. In contrast, the aphasic patient on any severity level may be impaired semantically, syntactically, and phonologically (except the Wernicke's aphasic, whose phonology is mostly intact), but may retain pragmatic behavior that is socially appropriate.

Gewirth, Shindler, and Hier (1984) studied the word associations of aphasia and dementia patients and found that production of syntagmatic responses (those less complex in language and usually elicited by verbs and adverbs) seems relatively resistant to deterioration in dementia or aphasia. However, production of paradigmatic responses (those more complex in language and usually elicited by nouns and adjectives) becomes progressively less efficient, and consequently more random (idiosyncratic) responses emerge in dementia than in aphasia.

Bayles, Tomoeda, and Caffrey (1982) suggest that a language test battery for dementia should assess the psychological and linguistic functions of learning, recent memory, remote memory, associative thought, orientation, ability to abstract, visual-spatial reasoning, expressive and receptive syntactic, phonologic, semantic, and pragmatic skills, verbal fluency, and verbal reasoning. These authors suggest specific test items for assessing these functions in addition to noting several radiographic procedures used by physicians, most notably the CAT (computerized axial tomography) scan, the PET (positron emission tomography) scan, and the rCBF (regional cerebral flow) measurement. Cummings and Benson (1983) offer additional information on differential diagnosis (pp. 10–14), assessment of mental status and language (pp. 15–34), and the use of laboratory procedures (pp. 285–307) for dementia.

With diagnosis in mind, Halpern, Darley, and Brown (1973) found that the group with generalized intellectual impairment was differentiated from the other groups (aphasia, confused language, and apraxia of speech) by impairment of reading comprehension and, to a lesser extent, auditory retention span. Relevance, however, was not subnormal. The neurologic data showed that the general intellectual impairment was of slow onset and long duration, associated with predominately diffuse lesions and caused by degeneration.

Deal, Wertz, and Spring (1981) replicated the above study, and they were able to pick out the aphasic patients (17 of 21), but had considerably less success in classifying the patients with the generalized intellectual impairment (only 8 of 15). However, when they used all the data—biographical, medical, and behavioral—all patients, aphasic as well as those with generalized intellectual impairment, were diagnosed correctly. Those authors, along with Wertz (1982), who used PICA data in his study, feel that aphasia can be differentiated from the language of generalized intellectual impairment.

Therapy

It is generally known that speech and language therapy or other treatments will not provide long-term improvement in the patient with generalized intellectual impairment. However, speech and language therapy can help the patient (and the family) to communicate maximally, within the scope of her limited abilities.

Therapy for generalized intellectual impairment should help orient the patient to time and place in a concrete manner. This can be achieved through the use of visual aids such as calendars, a blackboard for large words and simple drawings, and poster cards or large uncluttered pictures.

The clinician should determine what functions the patient will utilize in daily activities. This can be done by making grocery shopping lists, putting foods in categories, identifying the locations and names of supermarkets; practicing money concepts coupled with simple arithmetic; reading bus schedules (time, destinations, simple arithmetic); performing simple cooking activities (measuring with quarts, pints, pounds, ounces); setting clocks and timers (seconds, minutes, hours); and using the telephone for work on numbers in sequence and memory.

The clinician can try to help orient the patient to family placement and relationships by using real family names. Vocabulary should be concrete and centered around everyday activities. Participation in social situations should be encouraged to stimulate mental activity. Bayles, Tomoeda, and Caffrey (1982) point out that the family and caretakers can make many modifications in the way they communicate with the patient that will facilitate the comprehension and retention of information. Rate of speech, level of syntactic complexity, and the mode of linguistic input may all affect the patient's comprehension. Verbal analogies, fragmented discourse, humor, sarcasm, use of indefinite referents, conversation involving more than two individuals, and open-ended questions are the types of language that are hardest for the dementia patient.

In addition, those authors suggest counseling the family to (1) maintain a simple routine; (2) maintain a constant environment (dressing, eating, etc.); (3) be consistent; (4) minimize distractions; (5) provide indirect orientation to time and place (calendars, clocks, etc.); (6) provide memory aids (pictures of family members, etc.); (7) expect the patient to deny the problem; (8) expect the affected individual to become anxious; (9) simplify verbal interactions; (10) expect a change in the patient's condition if there is a major change in lifestyle; (11) avoid arguing with the affected individual; and (12) dispense the patient's medication and make sure the patient eats and exercises properly.

In summation, generalized intellectual impairment can be differentiated from aphasia. Whereas the aphasic has an uneven disturbance of all the modalities, the GII patient has an even impairment affecting all modalities. These patients have a bland, benign, noncaring attitude and are generally not frustrated when they miss easy questions. Not only does GII affect all the modalities but it can cut across into memory, judgment, thinking, and abstracting abilities. Emotional lability, at times, can cause the patient to go from a benign attitude to a highly irascible state. Generally, their responses become less relevant as the condition progresses.

The Language of Confusion

The language of confusion is a part of a condition in which the patient's responsiveness to his environment is impaired. The behavior indicates that the patient is less able to recognize and understand the environment than in the normal state. Clearness of thinking and accuracy of remembering are impaired. The patient usually manifests a disorientation of time and place, confabulations, inability to follow directions, bizarre and irrelevant responses, and unawareness of the inappropriateness of his responses (Darley, 1964, pp. 38–39; Halpern, Darley, & Brown, 1973; Mayo Clinic, 1964, p. 234; Wertz, 1978, pp. 1–101; 1984a, pp. 1–77).

Symptoms

Geschwind (1967) describes the syndrome of "nonaphasic misnaming" that typically occurs in disorders that diffusely involve the nervous system, especially when the disturbance comes on fairly rapidly.

Characteristically the errors tend to "propagate." Thus the patient, if asked where she is, may say "In a bus," and may continue by identifying the examiner as the bus driver, those around her as passengers, and her bed as one being used by the driver for resting. It is usually obvious once a sequence of questions is asked that ordinary aphasic misnaming is readily ruled out. Thus in aphasic misnaming there is no tendency to "propagation," although perseveration (i.e., repetition of the same incorrect word) occurs frequently.

The "connected" or "propagated" character of the errors may show up particularly in relation to the hospital and the patient's illness. He may call the hospital a "hotel," the doctors "bellboys," and the nurses "chambermaids," and will not accept correction.

One feature that often characterizes nonaphasic misnaming is that spontaneous speech is usually (but not invariably) normal despite gross errors in naming. In aphasia, errors in confrontation naming are almost always accompanied by a disturbance in spontaneous speech in which word-finding pauses, empty phrases, semantic or adequacy errors, and circumlocutions appear.

Stengel (1964) has stated that people in confusional states, when called upon to name objects, do not respond in the same way as aphasics, who say, "I know what it is, but I can't find the word." Confused patients boldly and sometimes recklessly improvise and produce words on the spur of the moment. These words may show effects of perseveration, slang, and other associations. They may contain references to certain aspects of the correct concept. The words produced may show a creative inventiveness. Occasionally they embody references to the patient's personal problems. The patients show no awareness of error and, when told to think again, insist that they are right. These responses, which have been called nonaphasic misnaming, are invariably associated with a more general change in behavior, whereby perception and motivation are altered. The disturbance of motivation is particularly obvious in relation to the task of naming and definition. These patients do not seem to care whether they obtain an accurate correspondence between the object and its generally accepted verbal representation. They disregard the function of language as a code behavior and of communication. They are either incapable of this effort or unwilling to make it.

Weinstein, Lyerly, Cole, and Ozer (1966) compared 18 jargon aphasics with 26 standard aphasics. Jargon consisted of phonetic distortions, mispronounced words, neologisms, standard English words put together in meaningless sequence, and sentences seemingly irrelevant to the subject under discussion. Jargon subjects had bilateral brain involvement and showed confabulation, particularly about the onset of the illness as the reason for coming to the hospital; disorientation for place and time; unawareness of errors; and lack of any catastrophic response. In the course of clinical improvement, the jargon was replaced by confabulations and the forms of idiomatic speech such as clichés, puns, and malapropisms. The greater the frequency of such verbalizations, the less was the degree of anxiety and overt concern. It seems that the jargon aphasia of the study by Weinstein, Lyerly, Cole, and Ozer (1966) and the nonaphasic misnaming as described by Geschwind (1967) and Stengel (1964) either are the same as confused language or resemble it.

In a study by Chedru and Geschwind (1972), 24 patients with metabolic or toxic disorders of rapid onset, and without focal brain lesion, were selected as "confused" on the basis of an alteration of attention. They were given a short neuropsychological examination, their performances being compared to those of 10 controls and to their own after recovering from confusion.

The following disorders were observed: disturbances of mood and behavior, disorientation, and unconcern toward illness; mild word-finding difficulties, tendency toward verbal paraphasias in repetition and reading tests, slowing of verbal fluency, and marked dysgraphia; mild spatial disturbances (right-left recognition), constructional apraxia, disturbances in finger recognition and in calculation, and memory defect. Most of the disorders disappeared completely after the acute confusional state cleared up.

Groher (1977) studied the memory and language skills of 14 patients who had suffered closed head trauma. He found that initially his subjects manifested both aphasic (a reduced capacity to interpret and formulate language symbols) and confused (faulty short-term memory, mistaken reasoning, inappropriate behavior, poor understanding of the environment, and disorientation) language skills. After a period of 1 month, both language and memory skills improved significantly. Continued improvement was made after 1 month and up to 4 months in both language and memory abilities, although deficits were still present in both areas at 4 months.

In a study of a single patient with the language of confusion, Drummond (1984) found that a monologue context ("Tell me how you would fry an egg") was more effective for observing linguistic irrelevancy than picture description. The monologue context provides a topic and requires the speaker to introduce different referents, expand on each of these referents, and then arrange them in a temporal hierarchy utilizing the past, present, and future dimensions. She also found that total utterances and impaired topic-focus organization were probably the most valid variables for describing linguistic irrelevancy. Both of these factors diminish progressively with physiological recovery.

From the studies cited, it is obvious that among the language skills the factor of impairment of relevance is a key differentiating point. In working with a confused language patient, I found the following to be typical examples of irrelevant responses. "A measure of violence" was given as the definition for *bargain*. "Should watch out for mail boxes, should watch out for people, should watch out for papers" was a response to the question of what three things every good citizen should do.

Etiology

The language of confusion can be caused by head injury, subarachnoid hemorrhage, rapidly increasing intracranial pressure, drug intoxication, withdrawal symptoms, acute infections, tumors, uremia, hepatic failure, and other types of metabolic disorders. The lesions are diffuse or disseminated. Although closed head injury can cause a number of speech and language disturbances (Hagen, 1984, pp. 245–281; Levin, 1981, pp. 427–433; M. Sarno, 1980), confused language is a common characteristic. From a medical point of view, Brosin (1967) sums up confusion as a disorder caused by reversible, temporary, diffuse disturbance in brain function. It is usually brief but may be prolonged up to 1 month or longer. It may end in health and cure, death, or chronic disease.

Diagnosis

In testing for confused language, the same procedures can be used as those described in testing for a generalized intellectual impairment. These can be added to any aphasia battery.

Darley (1964, pp. 38–39) sums up testing for confused language with the following considerations:

1. Is the patient oriented in space and time? Confused patients are frequently disoriented.
2. How well does the patient stay in contact with the examiner? The confused patient may unpredictably wander away from the conversation and engage in a colloquy upon some irrelevant subject. The confused patient may respond well to specific questions and discrete tasks but will "wander away" when given more freedom in response, as when asked open-ended questions or when required to explain proverbs or the functions of objects.
3. How aware is the patient of the inappropriateness of his responses? The confused patient tends to show clearly that he thinks he is "making sense," even when his responses are inadequate and irrelevant.
4. How well structured are the patient's responses? The confused patient may demonstrate normal sentence structure, whereas the content of the sentences is inappropriate.

Some of the linguistic, psychological, medical, and motor ability tests for assessing brain damage have been reviewed by Bayles, Tomoeda, and Caffrey (1982) and Levin (1981, pp. 423–463). Many of these can be used for evaluating the patient demonstrating confused language. In addition, Chedru and Geschwind (1972) offer some scoring criteria for evaluating the confused patient, and Cummings and Benson (1983, pp. 12–14) provide information on the differential diagnoses of acute confusional state and dementia.

The findings of the following studies can be used as an aid in the language diagnosis. The language findings of the study by Halpern, Darley, and Brown (1973) study indicated that the group with confused language was differentiated from the other groups (aphasia, generalized intellectual impairment, and apraxia of speech) by impairment in reading comprehension, writing words to dictation, and relevance. The neurologic data showed that the confused language was of sudden onset and short duration, associated with multiple focal lesions or mixed focal and diffuse lesions, and caused by trauma as often as by all other causes combined.

Studying a single patient, Mills and Drummond (1980) found that naming ability could be used as a discriminating factor between the language of confusion and that of aphasia. The factors of error rate and response time in naming tasks were more variable in the patient with the language of confusion than in aphasic patients. The greatest error rate and the longest response time took place in the early stages of recovery in the patient with confused language. In the latter stages of recovery, error rate and response time were close to normal. The aphasic patients were consistent throughout this time period. A greater percentage of semantically unrelated responses were found in the responses of the patient with confused language than those in the aphasic group.

Therapy

Therapy for the confused language patient tends to follow the same format as the therapy described for the patient with a generalized intellectual impairment. Therapy for the confused language patient would have to be quite structured and should be given as often as possible. At each session (preferably lasting 1 hour), the clinician should work on making the patient aware of the month, day, and year of that particular day as well as aware of the actual time and location of the therapy.

All the materials introduced to the patient should be actual concrete objects. The therapist should work on developing the patient's ability to name a given object, then to make specific comments about the particular object in question. Work should focus on basic attributes of a given object such as color, shape, size, weight, and texture. One-word fill-in type answers should be required to open-ended sentences (i.e, "This _____ is the color _____"). The patient should use a simple sentence to describe each attribute of the subject. Initially, each sentence response can be cued by saying, "Now, tell me about the _____ color," etc. The name of the object should be contained in the response, along with a specific attribute. The therapist should ask the patient to "tell me one thing about this _____" and work up to "tell me all you know about this _____." The patient should be required to give several of the previously worked-on attributes in sentence form as the correct response. This therapeutic procedure can be followed to build up a repertoire of nouns for the patient.

Pictures of the nouns used previously can be introduced as the first step in developing the patient's ability to deal relevantly on an abstract level. It is helpful to be optimistic and hope for maximum carryover. Upon introducing each picture, the clinician asks the patient to "tell me all you know about the picture." Depending on the moment of carryover, as evidenced by the type of response given by the patient, the patient's attention is directed to the specific picture at hand. She is helped to zero in on the attributes of the object in the picture so as to give a relevant response in reference to the specific object (picture).

The patient can be asked such questions as "What does this do? How does this work? What would you use this for?" in an effort to broaden the patient's amount of verbal output while still attempting to keep the patient focused on a specific object. Such questions are broad enough to let the patient have some freedom in verbal expression, yet specific enough to require a particular response.

Initially, the questions and responses should be as succinct as possible so as not to tax the patient. The next step would be short, simple conversations with the patient. This task is accomplished by gradually increasing the complexity of the verbalizations. Each time the patient demonstrates that he understands the particular level of syntactic and grammatic structure, the clinician moves to the next level and observes the patient's responses. Of course, if the patient's ability to function and respond appropriately cannot be developed, the verbalizations must be confined to the level at which the patient can function maximally.

Several techniques can be used to prevent or at least to limit the amount of irrelevant verbiage by the patient when a given stimulus requires a specific response. Initially, the therapist asks the patient to stop talking or uses a "time-out" procedure whenever the patient's response becomes irrelevant and wordy. As a last resort and only with selected patients, the therapist can leave the room upon a wordy, irrelevant response and reenter the room when the patient has stopped talking. Although the patient might object to the criticism of his responses and deny that he is in error, the therapist must convince the patient this judgment of his responses is the criterion measure and is geared solely for his benefit. It is important to establish a relationship in which the patient will place his trust in the therapist's judgment of his responses.

In summation, patients with confused language exhibit bizarre responses, irrelevant answers, confabulation, and propagation. They have a disorientation to time and space. Many times, their language structure is proper, but thought and content are improper. They are not communicating with their listener and show no insight or awareness of their inappropriate responses. Because of their irrelevant responses, they can at times resemble the patient with severe auditory comprehension deficit. However, the latter will do much better through the other modalities, whereas the confused language patient will be consistently bizarre or irrelevant regardless of modality.

The Language of Schizophrenia

In recent years, attention has been directed toward differentiating communication disorders in cerebrally involved populations (see, for example, Halpern, Darley, & Brown, 1973; Obler & Albert, 1981, chap. 6; Wertz, 1978, pp. 1–101; 1984a, pp. 1–77). Efforts have also been made to distinguish noncerebrally involved schizophrenic populations from nonschizophrenic cerebrally involved ones (see, for example, Cohen et al., 1977; Critchley, 1964; DiSimoni, Darley, & Aronson, 1977; Gerson, Benson, & Frazier, 1977; Halpern & McCartin-Clark, 1984). Information on whether a patient has the language of schizophrenia as opposed to the other communication disorders can be useful, for it helps to determine whether speech-language therapy is recommended and which kind of therapy is applicable. For example, therapy for the aphasic patient involves language training, whereas therapy might be contraindicated when the language of schizophrenia alone is diagnosed. Moreover, with psychiatric patients, conventional or traditional forms of therapy might be indicated but with certain modifications.

Another point to consider is that an overlapping or similar language symptom would require different approaches to therapy if that symptom is placed within a properly diagnosed syndrome. For instance, a semantic or adequacy error committed by an aphasic patient might take different forms of amelioration than one committed by a schizophrenic patient. To correct that type of error, the aphasic patient would most likely benefit from "stimulation-association" therapy and less likely benefit from "socialization" therapy. For the schizophrenic patient it would most likely be the reverse.

Information that differentiates the other communication disorders from the language of schizophrenia can further be used in detecting cerebral involvement in schizophrenic patients who were previously diagnosed as having no cerebral involvement. For example, some psychotic patients, because of their illness and long-term institutionalization, fall into a very noncommunicative routine. These individuals might suffer a slight stroke or other cerebral involvement and go undetected because of their seclusive institutional lifestyle. Language evaluation items that differentiate the other communication disorders from the language of schizophrenia might discover those who would otherwise go undetected.

The literature (see, for example, the reviews by Alpert, 1981, chap. 17; Darby, 1981, chap. 13; DiSiomoni, Darley, & Aronson, 1977; Hoffman, Kirstein, Stopek, & Cicchetti, 1982; Muller-Suur, 1981, chap. 16; and Ostwald, 1981, chap. 15) has indicated that the language of schizophrenia can contain numerous disturbances such as abnormal prosody, poor use for informational purposes, preoccupation with certain themes, stylized and quaint construction, disorientation, and confabulations, and fewer and more idiosyncratic word associations that that of normal individuals. Schizophrenic language varies with the situation (Rochester, 1980; Rochester & Martin, 1979) with emotionally tinged words (Richman, 1968), or with eomtionally negative topics (Salzinger, Portnoy, Feldman, & Patenaud-Lane, 1980, pp. 93–113). It can be relatively free of disorder syntax and most likely have simplified syntactic structures in its setences (Shapiro, 1979, p. 57; Wykes & Leff, 1982). Schizophrenic language can be influenced negatively by long-term institutionalization (Wynne, 1963). Recently, Chaika (1982) has postulated that the diverse errors in schizophrenic language are due to random or erroneous triggering of sounds and words and inappropriate preseverations.

The literature also notes that the language of some schizophrenic patients is paraphasic (Weinstein, 1956), neologistic (Weinstein, 1956; Whitehorn & Zipf, 1943), agrammatic and perseverative (Herbert & Waltensperger, 1980), and intermittently aphasic (Chaika, 1974, 1977; Hoffman & Sledge, 1984), thus resembling the language of aphasic patients. Others find that the language of schizophrenia is no different from that of aphasia (Chapman, 1966; Fish, 1957; Rumke & Nijdam, 1958). Finally, another body of opinion is that schizophrenia can be differentiated from aphasia (Benson, 1973; 1979, pp. 6, 89; Cohen et al., 1977; Critchley, 1964, 1970, pp. 349–351; Darley, 1982; Darley & Spriestersbach, 1978, p. 89; DiSimoni, Darley, & Aronson, 1977; Gerson, Benson, & Frazier, 1977; Halpern & McCartin-Clark, 1984; Karanth, 1981; Stengel, 1964, pp. 285–289; Wertz, 1978, pp. 1–101; 1984a, pp. 1–77) and from a generalized intellectual impairment, apraxia of speech, and the language of confusion (Darley, 1982; DiSimoni, Darley, & Aronson, 1977; Wertz, 1984a, pp. 1–77).

Symptoms

There is general agreement that schizophrenia is a disorder that affects the total personality in all aspects of its functioning. While not all patients show the same range in magnitude of disturbance, with even the same patients' symptoms varying from time to time, the striking feature of this disorder is that it permeates every aspect of the individual's functioning (Bemporad & Pinsker, 1974).

Day and Semrad (1978, pp. 199–241) point out that most schizophrenia begins in the mid-teens and continues at a high level of incidence until the mid-fifties. More women than men become schizophrenic. Married people are less susceptible than those who are single, separated, or divorced. Schizophrenia may affect the patient's perceptions, thoughts, affect, will, speech, motor control, and social behavior. These effects are briefly described as follows:

1. Perceptual disorders. Hallucinations, sense perceptions without related external stimuli, are most frequently auditory but may be visual, olfactory, or gustatory.

2. Cognitive or thought disorders. Schizophrenic delusions are false beliefs not subject to change by reason or experience.

3. Disorders of affect. Most schizophrenic patients express their feelings less frequently and less intensely than normal people, so that they appear indifferent or apathetic (emotional shallowness).

4. Volitional disorders. The schizophrenic patient's ambivalence and negativism and fears of the destructiveness of negative wishes impair or paralyze the will. Ambivalence is more intense than that of normals because it serves as a mechanism to deny pain and to avoid dealing with conflicts.

5. Verbal disorders. The schizophrenic patient's language tends to be excessively concrete yet privately symbolic. It can be incoherent, neologistic, mute, monosyllabic, echolalic, senselessly repetitive of words or phrases, stilted, and grotesquely quaint.
6. Motor disorders. Although motor activity is generally reduced in schizophrenics, extreme excitement that causes an increase in motor activity may occur, or motion may become awkward.
7. Disorders of social behavior. Withdrawal ranges from intense shyness to outright reclusiveness. There is disturbance in the capacity to experience pleasure, poor social competence, poor self-image, and poor cleanliness and dressing habits. Social amenities are poor.

Etiology

Although it is not clear what causes schizophrenia, four major factors contribute to each individual's clinical picture. Lehman (1967, pp. 593–598) and Day and Semrad (1978, pp. 199–241) outlined four areas of etiological research in schizophrenia: the genetic or inherited factor; the biochemical factor, or the possibility of a toxic factor that may be the result of an innate metabolic error. The psychodynamic factor, or the effects of early psychic trauma; and the social factor, or the role of the patient's disturbed family structure.

Diagnosis

Part of a diagnostic session might also involve differentiating the language of schizophrenia from other neurogenically caused communication disorders. Darley (1979, pp. 192–193) has pointed out that no single test differentiates aphasia from all the other disorders. However, he does cite research that shows how the PICA (Porch, 1971) might differentiate aphasia from apraxia of speech, malingering, and the language of bilateral involvement. A study by Horsfall (1972) found that PICA data showed schizophrenic subjects to be less severe than aphasic or bilaterally damaged patients. Wertz (1984a, p. 30) reanalyzed the Horsfall data and found that when performance is equated for severity in the three groups, there is little that differentiates schizophrenic patients from the other two groups. In a study by Cohen et al. (1977), a German version of the Sklar Aphasia Scale (Sklar, 1966) was used to differentiate between the language of aphasia, nonaphasia brain damage, schizophrenia, and normals.

With an eye toward diagnosis, the language of schizophrenia data from the Halpern and McCartin-Clark (1984) study was compared with the language data (Halpern, Darley, & Brown, 1973) of subjects with a generalized intellectual impairment, confused language, and apraxia of speech. This comparison revealed that although very close, subjects with a generalized intellectual impairment showed more impairment in auditory retention span, naming, and syntax than subjects with the language of schizophrenia. Subjects with confused language will be more impaired in reading comprehension, syntax, naming, relevance, writing words to dictation, and general overall language ability than subjects with the language of schizophrenia. Subjects with apraxia of speech will be more impaired in syntax, more nonfluent, and less impaired in relevance than subjects with the language of schizophrenia.

It seems that normal naming and syntactic ability of the schizophrenic group differentiates them from the above cerebrally involved groups, except for the apraxic subjects, where only syntactic ability differentiated them.

DiSimoni, Darley, and Aronson (1977) found that much impaired relevance and virtually unimpaired adequacy, naming, and syntax in their schizophrenic subjects differentiated them from the above cerebrally impaired groups. They found that schizophrenic subjects perform more poorly in nearly all categories as the duration of the illness increases. This suggests that as they age, their performance probably deteriorates first in the direction of the pattern shown by confused patients and ultimately toward the pattern shown by subjects with generalized intellectual impairment.

As stated earlier, the Halpern and McCartin-Clark (1984) study found that the language categories of strongest differentiating value were writing words to dictation, naming, syntax (where aphasic subjects were more impaired in all three), and relevance (where schizophrenic subjects were more impaired). DiSimoni, Darley, and Aronson (1977) found that aphasic subjects given similar tests to the schizophrenic subjects in their study typically have far less difficulty with relevance and have most difficulty with adequacy. The discrepancy between the two studies involving the language data of schizophrenic subjects using the same test battery is in the response category of adequacy.

In the Halpern and McCartin-Clark (1984) study, adequacy fell in the moderate range of impairment for both groups of subjects and was not deemed a differentiating factor. That language variable was found to be in the normal range and a differentiating factor by DiSimoni, Darley, and Aronson (1977) and to be rarely impaired by Gerson, Benson, and Frazier (1977). There is the possibility that many of the schizophrenic subjects in the Halpern and McCartin-Clark (1984) study suffer additionally from what is known as institutional neurosis. This condition, which is characterized mostly by apathy and sometimes a stereotyped posture and gait, affects individuals who are incarcerated in an institution for 2 years or longer. The probable causes of this condition are loss of contact with the outside world; enforced idleness and loss of responsibility; bossiness of medical and nursing staff; loss of friends, possessions, and personal effects;

drugs; ward atmosphere; and loss of prospects outside the institution. Since many of the above factors might interfere with the semantic or relational aspects of language, this may account for their findings. The mean length of institutionalization for their subjects was 6 years and 9 months, and 59 subjects were receiving drug therapy for their conditions. Karanth (1981) agrees with those results and states that the greatest overlap between aphasic and schizophrenic linguistic disabilities occurs in the area of semantics. She noted that both aphasic and schizophrenic patients may have difficulty in discriminating items within semantic categories such as colors, body parts, and items of furniture.

In the Halpern and McCartin-Clark (1984) schizophrenic group, length of institutionalization and speaking (especially adequacy and naming) were positively correlated, indicating that the longer one is institutionalized, the more speaking (especially adequacy and naming) errors one will produce. This finding agrees with Wynne (1963), who stated that schizophrenic language can be influenced by long-term institutionalization.

Many utterances of the schizophrenic patient resemble the adequacy errors of the aphasic patient. Although the end product, an adequacy error, is the same, in the aphasic patient it seems to be part of a word-finding disturbance (a linguistic inaccessibility), whereas in the schizophrenic patient it seems to be due to the underlying thought disorder, a lack of stimulation or socialization, and not caring. Apparently if the thought disorder component takes control, a bizarre response will be produced. If the lack of stimulation or socialization and the not-caring components take over, an adequacy error is produced. Critchley (1964) has indicated that one of the earliest and most fundamental purposes of language is to oprient (socialize) the individual within the community. The results of the Halpern, Darley, and Brown (1973) and Halpern and McCartin-Clark (1984) studies show that adequacy problems were the most common or least differentiating language symptoms of all the groups tested.

During a screening procedure, the clinician can engage the patient in open-ended conversation (i.e., "What did you have for lunch?") and have her name objects at hand, write several words from dictation, and follow directions through reading and auditory commands. Whether screening or going through a full battery, the clinician should use the medical data on the patient to help with a speech and language diagnosis.

In testing for the language of schizophrenia, any of the tests previously described for aphasia can be used. The clinician should concentrate on the less structured or more open-ended portions, such as defining words and proverbs, explaining three things that every good citizen should do, responding to an action picture, or elaborating a typical day. The time and place orientation and general information questions previously described in the testing discussion of a generalized intellectual impairment can be used.

Therapy

Speech and language therapy for the schizophrenic patient can consist of traditional or conventional approaches for whatever the communication problem is with room for adaptation to the individual patient. Some patients require highly structured situations while others might require loose and informal approaches. Reinforcements such as food and coffee work well. Therapy can be individual or group, and many times group therapy is provided so as not to drop the patient entirely.

Referrals are made by physicians and the hospital staff, and they should be directed by the speech pathologists in what to look for. Although progress is generally slower, speech and language therapy is beneficial because it raises the patient's communicative level in the institution and outside, if discharged. If mute, he is given some means of communication via sign language. In some cases, getting a patient to communicate can lead to release. At team meetings with the staff, it is most beneficial if the patient exhibits speech and language. Members of the team have been heard to say, "I didn't know he could speak that well." This can change the attitude toward the patient.

Patients will progress faster if they are helped to achieve carryover by assistance from the attendants. Attendants should be oriented by the speech pathologist on how to do this. For example, aides can ask questions related to everyday activities. Many times, if speech therapy stops, patients can revert to their previous stages. Often speech and language therapy is the only area in which any stimulation takes place. This stimulation can be in the form of socialization, which can be supportive in nature or in the conventional approaches, which work directly on their problem.

In addition to working with any coexisting aphasia, dysarthria, stuttering, or voice problem, in schizophrenic patients speech and language therapy can also try to overcome institutional neurosis, which is characterized by apathy and sometimes a stereotyped posture and gait. It is probably caused by incarceration in an institution for 2 years or longer and by the intake of drugs. Some speech pathologists who have worked in nonpsychiatric nursing homes see no difference when comparing those patients to patients in a psychiatric setting. They both have a form of institutional neurosis.

Audiological setups provide hearing aids and other aural rehabilitation procedures. Sign language can be taught to deaf patients, the mentally retarded, and the cerebral palsied. Patients are also taught alternate means of communication such as lipreading, descriptive gestures, and the use of communication boards.

Finally, as mentioned previously, it is quite common for psychiatric patients to have long-term ingestion of neuroleptic or antipsychotic medication. These drugs can produce a potentially irreversible disturbance of the central nervous system called *tardive dyskinesia*. The characteristics of this condition are abnormal movements within the oral musculature such as sucking and smacking noises, sudden protrusions and retractions of the tongue, rhythmic opening and closing of the mouth, and lateral jaw movements. Portnoy (1979) has pointed out that these symptoms are manifested in motor speech production as hyperkinetic dysarthria. Early detection by the speech pathologist and the audiologist of hyperkinetic dysarthria in such patients may play a critical role in the recognition of tardive dyskinesia during its reversible stages and thus help to prevent the onset of permanent damage to the central nervous system.

In a recent article, Darby, Simmons, and Berger (1984) found that 13 depressed subjects showed reduced stress, monopitch, and monoloudness, which is similar to hypokinetic dysarthria. They compared their results to the Parkinson subjects in the Darley, Aronson, and Brown (1975) study. They showed significant improvement after antidepressant medication treatment. The authors suggest that on the basis of the speech signs, a hypokinetic disturbance of the extrapyramidal system exists in depression.

In light of the above studies, it is seen that some psychotic patients may exhibit symptoms that resemble hyperkinetic dysarthria, whereas others may exhibit symptoms that resemble hypokinetic dysarthria. It is advisable to use the traditional or conventional methods, with room for individual adaptation of dysarthria therapy with these patients. Some suggestions for dysarthria therapy are mentioned later.

In summary, the language of schizophrenia can contain numerous disturbances, such as abnormal prosody, poor use of language for informational purposes, preoccupation with certain themes, stylized and quaint constructions, disorientation, and confabulations. It has been compared to aphasia, generalized intellectual impairment, and the language of confusion. The language of schizophrenia is different from those syndromes in that the overall language impairment is mild; the form and structure are good; and semantic, syntactic, and naming abilities are free of error while relevance is impaired. Generally, patients are noncaring and not frustrated about their problems in communication.

Apraxia of Speech

Apraxia of speech is an articulation disorder that results from impairment, due to brain damage, of the capacity to order the positioning of speech musculature and the sequencing of muscle movements for volitional production of phonemes and sequences of phonemes; but it is not accompanied by significant weakness, slowness, or incoordination of these same muscles in reflex and automatic acts (Darley, 1964, p. 36; Johns & Darley, 1970). This disorder can resemble a good deal of the oral expressive language behavior of the aphasic patient. For example, the phonemic groping of the apraxic patient can resemble the word-finding difficulty of the aphasic patient.

Symptoms

The studies cited below describe the symptoms of apraxia of speech. A major proportion of the material comes from Darley (1982, pp. 10–13), supplemented by the other literature listed.

1. Articulatory errors increase as the complexity of motor adjustment required of the articulators increases. Vowels evoke fewer errors than singleton consonants (Wertz, LaPointe, & Rosenbek, 1984, pp. 59–60). Of the singleton consonants, affricative and fricative phonemes evoke the most errors (Wertz, LaPointe, & Rosinbek, 1984, pp. 58–59). Most difficult of all are consonant clusters (Burns & Canter, 1977; Deal & Darley, 1972; Dunlop & Marquardt, 1977; Johns & Darley, 1970; LaPointe & Johns, 1975; Shankweiler & Harris, 1966; Trost & Canter, 1974; Wertz, LaPointe, & Rosenbek, 1984, pp. 58–59). Palatal and dental phonemes are significantly more susceptible to error than other phonemes classified according to place of production (LaPointe & Johns, 1975).

Repetition of a single consonant such as /puh/, /tuh/, or /kuh/ is ordinarily accomplished more easily than repetition of the sequence /puh-tuh-kuh/ (Rosenbek, Wertz, & Darley, 1973); on the latter task the patient is typically unable to maintain the correct sequence, even when he is repeatedly given a model to imitate. Klich, Ireland, and Weidner (1979) and Marquardt, Reinhart, and Peterson (1979) noted that apraxic patients made a systematic effort to reduce the articulatory complexity in the production of consonants. Keller (1984, pp. 221–256) also found that apraxic subjects tended to reduce the proportion of phoneme sequences (e.g., consonant clusters and diphthongs) and to increase the proportion of single consonants and single vowels in their speech. Wertz, LaPointe, and Rosenbek (1984, pp. 58–59) noted that a given sound can be correct in one position in a word but incorrect in another. They also noted that the production of easier consonants for more difficult ones is highly variable.

2. Initial consonants tend to be misarticulated more often than consonant phonemes in other positions (Hecaen, 1972; Shankweiler & Harris, 1966; Trost & Canter, 1974). Burns and Canter (1977) found that five patients with conduction aphasia and five with Wernicke's aphasia (mostly with posterior lesions) made what they called phonemic paraphasic errors more frequently in the final than in the initial position of words. However, Johns and Darley (1970) reported

that no single position in the word emerged as characteristically more difficult; LaPointe and Johns (1975) found error percentages for initial, medial, and final positions to be nearly equal; and Dunlop and Marquardt (1977) found phoneme position unrelated to occurrence of error. Klich, Ireland, and Weidner (1979) found that more substitutions were made in the initial word position. Wertz, LaPointe, and Rosenbek (1984, p. 62) concluded that sound position in a word may or may not have an influence on whether it will be produced accurately.

3. On repeated readings of the same material, apraxic patients demonstrate a consistency effect, tending to make errors at the same loci from trial to trial; they also demonstrate some adaptation effect, tending to make fewer errors on successive readings (Deal, 1974). The amount of reduction of errors is not great, varying from subject to subject.

4. Phonemes occurring with relatively high frequency in the language tend to be more accurately articulated than phonemes that occur less frequently (Trost and Canter, 1974; Wertz, LaPointe, & Rosenbek, 1984, pp. 62–63).

5. Numerous phonemic errors occur, including substitutions, omissions, additions, repetitions, and distortions, with a predominance of substitutions (Johns & Darley, 1970; LaPointe, 1969; LaPointe & Johns, 1975; LaPointe & Wertz, 1974; Trost, 1970; Wertz, LaPointe, & Rosenbek, 1984, pp. 52–53). Analysis of substitution errors made by apraxic patients according to the system of distinctive features indicates that the errors are variably related to the target sounds. Trost and Canter (1974), using a four-factor system, found that approximately 88% of the errors were one- or two-feature errors, most of the rest being three-feature errors. Slightly over half of the place errors observed were off target by one place, but about one third were off by two places. Martin and Rigrodsky (1974) found that more than 60% of the phonologic errors of their aphasic subjects were either one or two features away from target; they believed that the high degree of similarity between the error and the desired phoneme is not a haphazard occurrence of errors. They are related to the stimuli and may be reflective of either perceptual problems or memory decay.

LaPointe and Johns (1975) determined whether the substitutions made by their 13 apraxic patients were errors of placement, manner, or voicing, or combinations of these; they found that 38% of the errors were defective in two or more features and "bore little acoustic resemblance to the target sound." In their review of the literature, Wertz, LaPointe, and Rosenbek (1984, pp. 53–57) conclude that generally "apraxic patients are in the ballpark, most of the time. One or two phonetic feature errors predominate. Place and manner errors are common" (p. 56). They further concluded that apraxic patients generally "make more substitutions of voiceless consonants for voiced ones rather than the opposite" (p. 57).

6. When errors made by apraxic patients are analyzed with regard to sequential aspects, three types of errors are observed: anticipatory (prepositioning), reiterative (postpositioning), and metathesis (the order of two phonemes being reversed) (LaPointe & Johns, 1975). All 13 subjects in LaPointe and Johns' study produced some sequential errors, but the percentage of such errors relative to the total number of substitution and initiation errors was small (7%). Anticipatory errors outnumbered reiterative errors by a ratio of 6 to 1; metathesis of phonemes occurred rarely. Burns and Canter (1977) found more errors of phoneme sequencing among their "posterior" conduction aphasic patients and Wernicke's aphasic patients than Trost and Canter (1974) did among their "anterior" Broca's aphasic patients. Wertz, LaPointe, and Rosenbek (1984, pp. 57–58) noted that some patients display anticipatory, perseverative, and metathetic errors, most of which were anticipatory. However, all types of errors did not abound.

7. Apraxic patients display a marked discrepancy between their relatively good performance on automatic and reactive speech productions and their relatively poor volitional-purposive speech performance. "Words and phrases highly organized by practice and usage tend to sound normal" (Schuell, Jenkins, & Jimenez-Pabon, 1964, p. 265). Such islands of fluent, well-articulated speech appear in conversation, punctuated by episodes of effortful, off-target groping (Darley, 1969; LaPointe, 1969; LaPointe & Wertz, 1974; Wertz, LaPointe, and Rosenbek, 1984, pp. 65–66).

8. Imitative responses tend to be characterized by more articulatory errors than does spontaneous speech production. This holds true for single monosyllabic words as well as for material of greater length and complexity. Some patients display remarkably long latencies between the presentation of a stimulus word and their repetition of it (Schuell, Jenkins, & Jimenez-Pabon, 1964; Johns & Darley, 1970; Trost, 1970). On the other hand, Wertz, LaPointe, and Rosenbek (1984, pp. 66–67) found imitation to be better than spontaneous speech.

9. Articulation errors increase as length of words increases (Deal & Darley, 1972; DiSimoni & Darley, 1977; Wertz, LaPointe, & Rosenbek, 1984, pp. 63–64). As the patient produces a series of words with increasing number of syllables (*door, doorknob, doorkeeper, dormitory*), more errors are noted in all longer words. Such errors typically occur in the syllable common to all of the words, not just in the added syllables (Johns & Darley, 1970).

10. In oral reading of contextual material, articulatory errors do not occur at random; they are more frequent on words that carry linguistic or psychologic "weight" and that are more essential for communication (Deal & Darley, 1972; Hardison, Marquardt, & Peterson, 1977). The combination of word length and grammatical class has been found to be an especially important determinant of

the loci of errors. The difficulty level of initial phonemes also has a particularly negative effect on articulatory accuracy when combined with grammatical class. Grammatical class alone has not been found to be significantly related to occurrence of error (Deal & Darley, 1972; Dunlop & Marquardt, 1977; Wertz, LaPointe, & Rosenbek, 1984, p. 64). In general, when the complexity of a required response is increased, more errors occur. Any single characteristic may be insufficient to elicit error, but if characteristics are combined, their joint effect may be powerful enough to induce inaccuracies.

11. Correctness of articulation is influenced by mode of stimulus presentation (Johns & Darley, 1970; Trost & Canter, 1974). Patients tend to articulate more accurately when speech stimuli are presented by a visible examiner (auditory-visual mode) than when they imitate a stimulus presented by tape recorder (auditory mode) or spontaneously produce a word printed on a card (visual mode). Wertz, LaPointe, and Rosenbek (1984, p. 66) noted that the influence of stimulus mode is highly variable and depends on the individual patient.

12. Johns and Darley (1970) found that attainment of the correct articulatory target is facilitated more by repeated trials of a word than by increase in the number of stimulus presentations. Patients are more likely to be on target if they are given a model once and have three opportunities to imitate it than if they are permitted a single trial or are given three presentations of a model but only one trial to imitate it. LaPointe and Horner (1976) and Warren (1977) found that apraxic patients were extremely variable in their ability to improve on repeated trials. Wertz, LaPointe, and Rosenbek (1984, p. 67) observed that the process of repeated trials of a word to aid facilitation is highly variable and depends a good deal on the clinical process.

13. Accuracy of articulation in apraxic patients is not significantly influenced by a number of auditory, visual, and psychologic variables. For example, when patients perform a task under two conditions, one while observing themselves in the mirror and the other without such visual monitoring, the difference in the number of errors they produce is not statistically significant (Deal & Darley, 1972). Similarly, introduction of masking noise that prevents patients from hearing their own speech does not significantly alter the number of articulation errors they make (Deal & Darley, 1972; Wertz, LaPointe, & Rosenbek, 1984, pp. 68–69). Furthermore, articulatory performance is not improved when the patient is given an opportunity to delay an imitative response (Deal & Darley, 1972; Wertz, LaPointe, & Rosenbek, 1984, p. 68). Nor is articulatory accuracy influenced by the instructional set created in the speaker (Deal & Darley, 1972; Wertz, LaPointe, & Rosenbek, 1984, pp. 67–68). Patients do equally well (or poorly) in reading passages whether told that the passage is extremely easy, that it is loaded with hard words and phonemes and is extremely difficult, or that the degree of difficulty is unknown. Finally, incidence of errors is not sig-

nificantly influenced by imposing upon the patients speech and external auditory rhythm (metronome) (Shane & Darley, 1978; Wertz, LaPointe, & Rosenbek, 1984, pp. 68–69).

Recently, several studies (Collins, Rosenbek, & Wertz, 1983; Duffy & Garole, 1984, pp. 167–196; Hoit-Dalgaard, Murry, & Kopp 1983; Itoh & Sasanuma, 1984, pp. 135–165; Itoh et al., 1982 Kent & Rosenbek, 1982, 1983; Sands, Freeman, & harris, 1978; Shewan, Leeper, & Booth, 1984, pp. 197–220), using forms of instrumentation, have verified the temporal incoordination of apraxia subjects. Additional reviews concerning concepts of apraxia of speech can be found in Buckingham (1979, pp.271–30), Darley (1982, pp. 10–210, DeRenzi, Piezcuro, and Vignolo (1966), Kelso and Tuller (1981), Kent and Rosenbeck (1983), Rosenbeck, Kent, and LaPointe (1984, pp. 1–72), Wertz (1978, pp. 1–101), and Wertz, LaPointe, and Rosenbeck (1984).

Etiology

The etiology for apraxia of speech is brain damage—most likely a unilateral, left-hemisphere lesion involving the third frontal convolution (Kertesz, 1979, p. 187; Mohr, 1976, 1980; Mohr et al., 1978). Additional studies concerning etiology and site of brain lesion can be found in Deutsch (1984, pp. 113–134), Kertesz (1984, pp. 73–90), and Marquardt and Sussman (1984, pp. 91–112).

Diagnosis

In testing for apraxia of speech, the following procedures can be used along with the tests used in aphasia evaluation. The patient is asked to repeat sounds, syllables, words, and sentences after the examiner. For example, while looking for the symptoms described previously, the examiner asks the patient to do the following: (1) prolong /ah/; (2) prolong /ee/; (3) prolong /oo/; (4) repeat /puh/ rapidly; (5) repeat /tuh/ rapidly; (6) repeat /kuh/ rapidly; (7) repeat /puh-tuh-kuh/ rapidly; (8) repeat *snowman*; (9) repeat *gingerbread*; (10) repeat *impossibility*. Responses can be scored as accurate and immediate; accurate but delayed or acceptable overall pattern with defective amplitude, accuracy, force, or speed; and partial perseverative, irrelevant, or nil.

Patients can also be asked to respond out loud to pictures, read out loud a phonetically balanced passage (i.e., grandfather passage), and respond to standardized articulation tests.

A more formalized test called the Apraxia Battery for Adults (Dabul, 1979) checks for apraxia of speech by having the patient produce a timed diadochokinetic task, repeat words of increasing length, name pictures within a specific time period, read out loud, produce automatic speech by counting, and engage in spontaneous speech. A quantified scoring method is incorporated in the test.

Wertz, LaPointe, and Rosenbek (1984, pp. 98–103) describe their Motor Speech Evaluation, whose origin is spread throughout the literature. It is a screening tool that usually takes less than 20 minutes to administer. Scoring the test can be descriptive (e.g., "A" for apraxic productions, "P" for paraphasias, "D" for dysarthria, "U" for nondiagnostic errors, "O" for other errors, and "N" for normal responses). Or scoring can be multidimensional (e.g., utilizing the PICA 16-point scale). Or it can use narrow or broad phonetic transcription.

The tasks are traditional: (1) conversation; (2) vowel prolongation; (3) repetition of monosyllables /puh/, /tuh/, /kuh/; (4) repetition of a sequence of monosyllables like /puh-tuh-kuh/; (5) repetition of multisyllabic words; (6) multiple trials with the same word; (7) repetition of words that increase in length (*thick, thicken, thickening*); (8) repetition of monosyllabic words that contain the same initial and final sound (*mom, judge*, etc.); (9) repetition of sentences; (10) counting forward and backward; (11) picture description; (12) repetition of sentences used volitionally to determine consistency of production; and (13) oral reading.

Wertz, LaPointe, and Rosenbek (1984, pp. 103–107) further describe sound by position tests, the influence of stimulus modes, and procedures for scoring and determining severity. LaPointe (1982, pp. 370–400) suggests gathering information from the personal history, the nonspeech functions of the structures of speech, conversational and social interactive speech, and special speech tasks. In particular, he has noted methods of diagnosis involving repetition of syllables, imitating of single-syllable words, imitation of longer words, sentence imitation, reading aloud standard passages, and spontaneous speech. Recently, Wertz (1984b, pp. 257–276) described some of the difficulties in assessing apraxia of speech. He advocates using a comprehensive set of tasks sensitive enough to tap the ambiguous patient.

As an aid in diagnosis, the Halpern, Darley, and Brown (1973) language findings showed the prominence of the lack of fluency as the characteristic that distinguishes the apraxia of speech group from the other three groups (aphasia, generalized intellectual impairment, and confused language). The neurologic data showed that the apraxia of speech tended to be of sudden onset but variable duration, associated with anterior infarcts.

Prognosis

After reviewing the literature, Wertz, LaPointe, and Rosenbek (1984, pp. 142–145) have concluded that no significant variables influence prognosis in apraxia of speech. However, due to their own clinical experience and what the literature says, they do feel that particular patients might have a favorable prognosis. These patients have the following characteristics: are less than 1 month postonset; suffered a small lesion confined to Broca's area; have minimal coexisting aphasia; do not display significant oral, nonverbal apraxia; are in good health; and have the stamina for intensive treatment. They further feel (pp. 158–159) that the combination of education, counseling, and drill along with the patient's ability to learn, to generalize, and a willingness to practice enhances the prognosis for improved speech. They note that untreated apraxic patients do not reach the same competence as do those who are treated. Thus, the prognosis for functional recovery is poor without treatment, fair with treatment for the severe patient, and good with treatment for the moderate-to-mild patient.

Therapy

Darley, Aronson, and Brown (1975, pp. 270–271) suggest the following fundamental principles that underlie therapy for the motor speech disorders:

1. Compensation. The patient learns to make maximum use of the remaining potential and to "work around" the impairment that has altered his lifelong speech habits.
2. Purposeful activity. The patient learns to do on purpose what he had been doing automatically before. He must develop an awareness of where his articulators are and what they are doing, how word sequences fall into phrase groupings, how breath supply can be coordinated with the onset of speech effort and adjusted to the appropriate phrase units, and how his voice varies in loudness.
3. Monitoring. The patient learns to listen to himself talk, perhaps by listening to tape recordings of his speech performances from time to time, noting specific ways in which he falls short of his standard, whether in audibility, intelligibility, or emphasis.
4. An early start. The patient gets a head start in compensation, purposeful activity, and monitoring before his skills have deteriorated and before it becomes next to impossible to sustain the effort to speak well.
5. Motivation. The patient is reassured that his effort is worthwhile. The clinician plans a sensible sequence of activities, graduated in difficulty with an optimistic manner that encourages the patient to do his best.

Recently, Beukelman (1984a, pp. 101–103), Hartman, Day, and Pecora (1979), and LaPointe (1982, pp. 392–393) have reported on effectively utilizing these principles in treating patients with motor speech disorders. For clinical experience, Rosenbek (1984, pp. 49–56) has indicated that apraxia patients have a good prognosis for speech rehabilitation.

Rosenbek et al. (1973) and Wertz, LaPointe, and Rosenbek (1984, pp. 172–174) point out that therapy for apraxia of speech should concentrate on the disordered articulation and therefore differ from the language stimulation and audiotory and visual processing therapies appropriate to the aphasias or the dysarthrias (Wertz, LaPointe, Rosenbek, 1984, pp. 167–169), where multiple problems due to paralysis exist (e.g., strengthing exercises for a weak musculature would be appropriate in many dysarthric patients but is not called for in apraxia of speech). In genral, a variety of phonetic conditions affect articulatory accuracy of the speech patient in predictable ways.

These phonetic conditions are as follows: manner of articulation, where fricatives, affricatives, and consonant clusters are more likely to be in error than vowels, nasals, and plosives; phoneme position, where errors are more likely in initial than final phoneme; difficulty of initial phoneme, where the word is more likely to be in error if it begins with a fricative, affricative, or consonant cluster; distance between successive phonemes, where likelihood of error increases as distance between successive points of articulation within an utterance increases; word length, where errors increase as words increase in length; and word frequency, where errors occur more readily on rare than on common words. Trost and Canter (1974) found that phonemes with relatively high frequency tend to be more accurately articulated than those that occur less frequently. Therapeutic principles derived from the phonetic conditions described above should be considered when beginning therapy. A review and clinical application of many of these conditions can be found in Wertz, LaPointe, and Rosenbek (1984, pp. 180–202).

Articulatory accuracy in apraxia of speech is influenced by mode of stimulus (Johns & Darley, 1970; Trost & Canter, 1974). Johns and Darley (1970) found that auditory-visual stimulation is better than auditory or visual alone—visual in this instance referring to watching the clinician as she speaks. However, LaPointe and Horner (1976) found no differences in correct production among single and combined modes of stimulation. Deal and Darley (1972) found that apraxic patients do not achieve greater phonemic accuracy if they are allowed to monitor their own speech in a mirror.

Auditory training does not necessarily precede production when instituting therapy. The apraxic who is either pure or only mildly aphasic can show auditory perception difficulties, as Aten, Johns, and Darley (1971) have demonstrated, or can have little or no auditory perception problems, as Square (1981) has shown. Nor does therapy necessarily employ a motokinesthetic approach (manual manipulation of the articulators for correct production) because deficits in oral sensation and perception have been demonstrated (Rosenbek, Wertz, & Darley, 1973). Deutsch (1981) found that oral form identification deficits are not causally related to motor speech programming problems.

Therapy does emphasize the auditory and visual modalities, and especially the visual, because these clinically appear to be most potent in guiding the articulators. While it has not yet been experimentally confirmed, it appears that establishing or strengthening "visual memory" is most important to therapeutic success with the apraxic adult. The phonetic placement method of describing the correct manner and place of articulation and the correct voiced and voiceless components of phoneme production is useful. Rosenbek (1984, pp. 49–56) and Wertz, LaPointe, and Rosenbek (1984, pp. 174–178) further elaborate on the use of multimodality therapy procedures. Utilizing the general conditions mentioned above, Rosenbek et al. (1973) advocate an eight-step integral stimulation ("Listen to me and watch me") method as an approach to therapy with apraxic patients. In a later study, Deal and Florance (1978) further elaborate on this eight-step task continuum program.

Dabul and Bollier (1976) observe that the apraxic patient's most characteristic problem is the sequencing of speech sounds. They advocate the use of nonmeaningful syllable combinations in order to focus the patient's attention on the necessary phoneme sequencing and away from the decision on whether movements were voluntary or automatic. They found that mastery of volitional control over nonmeaningful syllable combinations leads to improved articulation of meaningful words. However, Rosenbek (1984, pp. 49–56) and Wertz, LaPointe, and Rosenbek (1984, p. 63) favor the use of meaningful stimuli because of its clinical success.

Sparks and Holland (1976) have reported success in using melodic intonation therapy (MIT) with nonfluent patients who exhibit relatively good auditory comprehension, frequent phonemic errors, and poor repetition skill. The intoned pattern is based on one of several speech prosody patterns that are reasonable choices for a given sentence, depending on the inference intended. The three elements are the melodic line, the rhythm, and points of stress. Through a gradual progression of carefully intoned sentences and phonemes, the patient is guided to normal prosody to aid speech return. A full discussion of this form of therapy can be found in Sparks (1981). Rosenbek, Hansen, Baughman, and Lemme (1974) and Yoss and Darley (1974) have found that various rhythmic techniques can be used to increase articulatory accuracy, whereas Shane and Darley (1978) found that auditory rhythmic stimulation (metronome) did not significantly improve articulatory accuracy.

Keith and Aronson (1975) described the use of singing. Rosenbek (1978, pp. 220–226) and Wertz, LaPointe, and Rosenbek (1984, pp. 238–248, 267–273) reviewed the use of gestural programs as an alternative mode of communication for the profoundly involved and as a supplemental mode (Rosenbek, 1984, pp. 49–56) in patients with severe involvement. Lane and Samples (1981) report the successful use of Blissymbols as a facilitory technique. Rosenbek (1978, pp.

220–226) also describes the use of instruments (binaural maskers, delayed auditory feedback devices, metronomes, and electromyographic feedback devices) as a means of slowing the rate, accenting stress patterns, and relaxing the speech musculature in the treatment of apraxia of speech. Wertz, LaPointe, and Rosenbek (1984, pp. 273–276) note the successful use of a pacing board in therapy.

Recently, Wertz (1984b, pp. 257–276) has reviewed and found in his own study that patients with aphaxia of speech do benefit from the types of therapy previously described. LaPointe (1984, pp. 277–286) provides some methods of evaluating success in therapy with these patients. Rubow, Rosenbek, Collins, and Longstreth (1982) note the effectiveness of vibrotactile stimulation coupled with auditory stress and rhythm cues with an apractic patient. Additional reviews and therapeutic techniques for apraxia of speech have been described by Darley, Aronson, and Brown (1975, pp. 280–285), Halpern (1981, pp. 347–360), Johns and LaPointe (1976, pp. 161–199), Rosenbek (1978, pp. 191–241), Rosenbek, Kent, and LaPointe (1984, pp. 1–72), and Rosenbek (1984, pp. 203–295).

Summing up, apraxia of speech can be described as a peculiar type of speaking problem. Those patients with pure apraxia of speech would not have any difficulty in any of the modalities except oral expression. They are highly inconsistent in their errors, have difficulty in getting started, and at times have the ability to give a correct production after a number of faulty attempts. Most of their trouble comes when asked to say something upon confrontation or command; they will have less difficulty when their speech is automatic or reflexive. Apraxia of speech is not a linguistic disturbance but rather a programming or transmissive problem. The language of these patients is relevant to the situation, and they will not exhibit bizarre responses. When in error, they will recognize it and show frustration in their efforts to correct themselves.

Dysarthria

The condition known as dysarthria can occur alone or can accompany other speech and language disorders. Abbs, Hunker, and Barlo (1983, pp. 21–56), Aronson (1980, pp. 77–115), Canter (1967), Froeschels (1943), Grewel (1957), Luchsinger and Arnold (1965), Netsell (1983, pp. 1–19; 1984, pp. 1–36), and Peacher (1950) have offered reviews and concepts concerning dysarthria. In a comprehensive study, Darley, Aronson, and Brown (1969a, 1969b, 1975) state that dysarthria is a collective name for a group of speech disorders resulting from disturbances in muscular control over the speech mechanism due to damage of the central or peripheral nervous system. Dysarthria designates an impairment in oral communication due to paralysis, weakness, or incoordination of the speech musculature. This disorder is in contrast to impairments due to damage to higher centers related to the faulty programming of movement and sequences of movements (apraxia of speech) and to the inefficient processing of linguistic units (aphasia).

Darley, Aronson, and Brown (1969a, 1969b, 1975) delineate six types of dysarthria, each with its own neurologic and speech characteristics. However, imprecise consonants were found in all or practically all of the subjects in all groups. An analysis of the misarticulations of adult dysarthric subjects can be found in Platt, Andrews, Young, and Quinn (1980b) and Platt, Andrews, and Howie (1980a). Monopitch, monoloudness, and harsh quality are also frequently observed in all groups. Although the overall rate was judged to be slower than average in every other neurologic group studied, the Parkinsonian group was unique in presenting what appears to be a faster than average rate or an impression of festination (acceleration during speaking). Recently, Portnoy and Aronson (1982) confirmed that spastic and ataxic dysarthric subjects had a significantly slower and more variable rate in repetition tasks than normals. Linebaugh and Wolfe (1984, pp. 199–205) found that ataxic and spastic dysarthric speakers had significantly longer mean syllable duration than did normal speakers.

Types of Dysarthria

The first type is described as *flaccid dysarthria* and is generally found in the neurologic disorder called bulbar palsy. All patients in this group displayed evidence of a lower motor neuron lesion, implicating motor units of the cranial nerves involved in speech (V, VII, IX–X, XII). The outstanding characteristics of flaccid dysarthria are hypernasality, nasal emission of air, and breathiness.

The second type is described as *spastic dysarthria* and is generally found in the neurologic disorder called pseudobulbar palsy. The patients constituting the pseudobulbar group present an upper motor neuron disorder, presumed to involve combined damage to the pyramidal system and to a portion of the extrapyramidal system, which both arise from the same motor cortex areas. Etiology may be multiple strokes, brain injury sustained in accidents, cerebral palsy, extensive brain tumors, encephalitis, multiple sclerosis, or progressive degeneration of the brain. The outstanding characteristics of spastic dysarthria are the harsh, strain-strangled voice, and low pitch.

The third type is described as *mixed dysarthria* and is generally found in the neurologic disorder called amyotrophic lateral sclerosis. In amyotrophic lateral sclerosis (ALS) there is progressive degeneration of both upper and lower motor neurons. One should expect the speech of patients with this disease to exhibit both bulbar (flaccid dysarthria) and pseudobulbar (spastic dysarthria) characteristics, truly a "mixed dysarthria." The outstanding characteristics of mixed dysarthria are the severe nature of hypernasality, breathy voice, and slow rate. Dworkin, Aronson, and Mulder (1980) found that dysarthric patients with ALS had lower tongue force and slower syllable repetitions than normal subjects. A negative correlation existed between tongue force and severity of articulation and syllable rate and severity of articulation in ALS. The problems of respiration and their effect upon the speech of ALS and other motor neuron disease patients can be found in Putnam and Hixon (1984, pp. 37–67).

Additional "mixed" types of dysarthria have been found in the neurologic disorders of multiple sclerosis (Darley, Aronson, & Brown, 1975; Darley, Brown, & Goldstein, 1972), which showed ataxic and spastic components; Wilson's disease (Berry, Darley, Aronson, & Goldstein, 1974; Darley, Aronson, & Brown, 1975), which showed ataxic, spastic, and hypokinetic components; and the Shy-Drager syndrome (Linebaugh, 1979), which showed ataxic, hypokinetic, and spastic components.

The fourth type is described as *hypokinetic dysarthria* and is generally found in the neurologic disorder called Parkinsonism. Common causes of Parkinsonism are encephalitis, degeneration of nerve cells due to aging or arteriosclerotic changes, repeated small injuries of the head, birth injuries and congenital diseases, exposure to certain toxins, and certain tranquilizing drugs. The outstanding characteristics of hypokinetic dysarthria are severe monopitch, monoloudness, and reduced stress. With many Parkinson patients, the administration of the drug L-dopa has brought about a lessening of these symptoms. Logemann, Fisher, Boshes, and Blonsky (1978) described the frequency of occurrence and the cooccurrence of speech and voice symptoms in 200 Parkinson patients. They classified these patients into five groups: Group 1 (45% of the patients)—with laryngeal dysfunction as their only vocal-tract symptom; Group 2 (13.5% of the patients)—with laryngeal and back-tongue involvement; Group 3 (17% of patients)—with laryngeal, back-tongue, and tongue-blade dysfunction; Group 4 (5.5% of the patients)—with laryngeal dysfunction, back-tongue involvement, tongue-blade dysfunction, and labial misarticulation; and Group 5 (9% of the patients)—with laryngeal dysfunction and misarticulations of the back tongue, tongue blade, lips, and tongue tip.

In a follow-up study, Logemann and Fisher (1981) found inadequate tongue elevation to achieve complete closure on stop plosives and affricates and inadequate close constriction of the airway in lingual fricatives. Recently, Kent and Rosenbek (1982) have given an acoustic description of the prosodic disturbances associated with Parkinsonian dysarthria. Hunker and Abbs (1984, pp. 69–100) have provided a phonological analysis of Parkinsonian tremors and their effect upon speech, and Weismer (1984, pp. 101–130) has further described the articulatory characteristics of 8 subjects with Parkinsonian dysarthria.

The fifth type is described as *hyperkinetic dysarthria* and is generally found in the neurologic disorders called dystonia and chorea. The common causes of dystonia and chorea are the same as described previously under Parkinsonism. The outstanding characteristics of hyperkinetic dysarthria are the distortion of vowels, alteration of loudness, excessive loudness variations, voice stoppages (dystonia), and the momentary interruption of any of the motor speech processes involved with respiration, phonation, articulation, hypernasality, and prosody (chorea).

As mentioned previously, Portnoy (1979) noted that tardive dyskinesia is manifested in motor speech production as hyperkinetic dysarthria. Recently, Golper, Nutt, Rau, and Coleman (1983) described the speech management program for 10 patients with focal cranial dystonia who showed a slow hyperkinetic dysarthria.

The sixth type is described as *ataxic dysarthria* and is generally found in neurologic cerebellar disorders. When the causative lesion – whether tumor, progressive degeneration, trauma, multiple sclerosis, toxicity from alcohol excess, strokes, or congenital conditions – involves both sides of the cerebellum and ataxia of both upper extremities is observed, ataxic speech is generally present. The outstanding characteristics of ataxic dysarthria are the irregular articulatory breakdown and the excessive and equal stress. In a recent study by Hirose, Kiritani, Ushijima, and Sawashima (1978), EMG findings showed physiological evidence of inconsistency in the articulatory movement of an ataxic dysarthric. This pattern seems to be compatible with the characteristic of irregular articulatory breakdown in ataxic dysarthria. Kent, Netsell, and Abbs (1979) have described the acoustic characteristics of 5 subjects with ataxic dysarthria, and Joanette and Dudley (1980) have described the general dysarthric and phonatory stenosis factors in 22 subjects with Friedreich's ataxia. Recently, Kent and Rosenbek (1982) provided an acoustic description of the prosodic disturbances associated with ataxic dysarthria. Murry (1984, pp. 79–89) has noted that Friedreich's ataxia involves more explosive speech than cerebellar ataxia. Phonatory characteristics are more bizarre in that there is a rough or harsh quality along with a strain-strangled quality.

Diagnosis

A systematic evaluation of dysarthria requires a sample of several types of speech and voice production. Darley, Aronson, and Brown (1975) suggest that a sample of conceptual speech can be elicited by having the patient tell about a picture representing a situation, or by having the patient read a standard paragraph of simple prose containing all the consonants and vowels of English as well as some consonant clusters. Patients can also respond to standardized articulation tests. Tikofsky and Tikofsky (1964) and Yorkston and Beukelman (1980) have proposed that dysarthrics read lists of words; based upon their intelligibility, the clinician can determine degrees of impairment. In a later study, Yorkston and Beukelman (1981a) found that speaking rate and speech intelligibility can distinguish mildly dysarthric from normal speakers.

Beukelman and Yorkston (1980a) also found that speech pathologists overestimated intelligibility of dysarthric speech because, it was hypothesized, of familiarity with the passage. In a later study, Yorkston and Beukelman (1983, pp. 155–163) found that familiarization with the dysarthric speaker did not increase intelligibility scores. Recently, Ansel, McNeill, Hunker, and Bliss (1983, pp. 85-106) looked at the relationship between the severity of intelligibility impairment and the verbal adjustments made by adult dysarthric subjects. Additional descriptions of intelligibility of dysarthric speakers can be found in Beukelman and Yorkston (1979) and Grunwell and Huskins (1979).

Assessment of Intelligibility of Dysarthric Speech (Yorkston and Beukelman, 1981b) is a tool for quantifying single-word intelligibility, sentence intelligibility, and speaking rate of adult and adolescent dysarthric speakers. Measures of speech intelligibility and speaking rate serve as an index of dysarthric severity, thus enabling the clinician to rank order different dysarthric speakers, compare performance of a single dysarthric speaker to normal performance, and monitor changing performance over time.

The Frenchay Dysarthria Assessment (Enderby 1983b) is another test that can be used for evaluation of dysarthria. This test is divided into 11 sections: Reflex, Respiration, Lips, Jaw, Palate, Larynx, Tongue, Intelligibility, Rate, Sensation, and Influencing Factors (hearing, sight, teeth, language, mood). The patient is asked to perform designated tasks (e.g "Say 'ah' for as long as possible" and "Count to twenty as quickly as possible") on eight of the sections. Scoring is based on a patient's second attempt at each task. A 9-point rating scale is used.

Netsell and Cleeland (1973) offered some techniques in the diagnosis of velopharyngeal dysfunction in dysarthric speakers. These techniques utilize simultaneous recordings of intraoral air pressure, rate of nasal air flow, and the speech signal. Some researchers have advocated the use of oral perception for diagnosis. Kent and Netsell (1975) and Simmons (1983, pp. 283–294) performed cineradiographic and spectrographic analysis to study the speech production of a subject who presented the classic neurological signs of cerebellar lesion and had speech characteristics similar to those that have been reported for ataxic dysarthria.

Recently, Barlow, Cole, and Abbs (1983) described a head-mounted lip-jaw movement transduction system for the study of motor speech disorders, and Barlow and Abbs (1983) further described the use of force transducers for the evaluation of labial, lingual, and mandibular motor impairments. Hixon, Putnam, and Sharp (1983) discuss the use of a kinematic procedure in measuring speech production in a patient with flaccid paralysis of the rib cage, diaphragm, and abdomen. O'Dwyer et al. (1983) note the use of EMG in evaluating the activity of orofacial and mandibular muscles of dysarthric subjects during nonspeech tasks.

In additional testing for dysarthria, the following procedures can be used along with the tests used in aphasia evaluation. The clinician should look for the symptoms described under each type of dysarthria and ask the patient to do the following: (1) prolong /ah/, /ee/, and /oo/ separately as long, as clearly, and as steadily as possible; (2) repeat /puh/ as rapidly as possible; (3) repeat /tuh/ as rapidly as possible; (4) repeat /kuh/ as rapidly as possible; and (5) repeat / puh-tuh-kuh/ as rapidly as possible. Perceptual evaluation of dysarthria utilizes the motor speech tasks listed for evaluating apraxia of speech. They include repetition of words and sentences. Evaluation can also include LaPointe's (1982, pp. 370–400) review of the assessment of the functioning of the valves in the point-place system. The valves in this system involve the muscles and structure of respiration, the larynx, the velum and velopharyngeal area, the tongue blade, the tongue tip, the lips, and the mandible.

For the severely dysarthric speaker, Owens and House (1984) and Shane and Bashir (1980) offer criteria for determining candidacy for an augmentative system. Included is a consideration of cognitive, oral reflex, language, motor, intelligibility, emotional, chronological age, previous therapy, imitative, and environmental factors. Beukelman and Yorkston (1980b), Coleman, Cook, and Meyers (1980), and Wilson and Antablin (1980) provide additional assessment procedures for nonvocal communication of severely dysarthric patients. Additional assessment procedures can be found in Collins (1984), DeFeo and Schaefer (1983, pp. 165–186), Enderby (1983a, pp. 109–119), Ludlow and Bossich (1983, pp. 121–153; 1984, pp. 163–195), and Yorkston, Beukelman, Minifie, and Sapir (1984, pp. 131–162).

In an effort to clairfy the distinction between dysarthria and apraxia of speech, Darley (1982, p. 13), Darley, Aronson, and Brown (1975, p. 251), Halpern (1978; 1980), Wertz (1978, p. 86), and Wertz, LaPointe, and Rosenbek (1984, pp. 127–129) state that generally dysarthria involves all speech levels (respiration, phonation, articulation, resonance, and prosody), while apraxia is primarily a disorder of articulation and prosody (maybe caused by compensatory behaviors). Usually dysarthria is characterized by distortion errors while apraxia is characterized by substitution errors. Dysarthric errors are probably more consistent than apraxic errors; however, mild dysarthria is probably less consistent than severe apraxia of speech. In apraxia of speech, neurologic examination reveals no significant evidence of slowness, weakness, incoordination, or alternation of tone of the speech musculature as in dysarthria.

Darley (1982, p. 13) and Darley, Aronson, and Brown (1975, p. 251) further note that at the onset of apraxia of speech, the patient may experience difficulty initiating phonation at will; once this difficulty passes, as it usually does in a few days, phonation and resonance are normal. In dysarthria, the articulatory errors are characteristically errors of simplification (distortions and omissions). In apraxia of speech, there is a preponderance of errors that must be considered complications of speech (substitutions of other phonemes, additions of phonemes, substitutions of a consonant cluster for a single consonant, repetitions of phonemes, and prolongations of phonemes).

Rosenbek, Kent, and LaPointe (1984, pp. 41-42) note that recent research has shown that more distortion errors have crept into the symptomatology of apraxia of speech. In spite of this, they state their clinical rule that dysarthria is the most likely diagnosis if a patient has a high proportion of relatively consistent distortions. Apraxia of speech is the likely diagnosis if distortions are mixed with what sound like substitutions, especially if such errors are relatively inconsistent.

Prognosis

Netsell (1984, pp. 23-26) has suggested six factors that influence treatment outcome with dysarthric patients:

1. Neurologic status and history. Bilateral subcortical or brain-stem lesions and degenerative diseases such as ALS offer the poorest prognosis. Love, Hagerman, and Taimi (1980) found that cerebral palsy subjects with more frequent dysphagic symptoms tended to present lower score of overall speech proficiency and poor articulation scores. Neurologic history should be observed to see if developmental (e.g., cerebral palsy) or acquired dysarthria is present. Treatment procedures geared specifically to the cause would offer a better prognosis.
2. Age. Persons experiencing neurological insults following early but incomplete development of the neocortical system (after age 2 or 3) might be expected to have, or to develop, better speech motor skills than those learned earlier. The implication is that intact reticulolimbic systems can support the more innate early motor skills. Younger children have a better chance to "grow out of" their lesions than adults. Elderly patients are negatively affected by age.
3. "Automatic" adjustments. In response to a lesion, "automatic" adjustments can be adaptive or maladaptive, intended or unintended, and reactive or

"obligatory" (always the same). Incorporating "automatic" adjustments that are useful and minimizing those that are not offer a better prognosis.

4. Treatment effects. Treatment, especially combined (speech, medical, physical, behavioral), is better than no therapy or noncoordinated therapy.
5. Personality and intelligence. Those who were optimistic and purposeful before injury have a better prognosis than those who were not. Understanding premorbid levels of intelligence should aid in therapy.
6. Support systems. Treatment is enhanced if support is given by "significant others" and if the prospects for making contributions to society, however modest, are realistic.

Therapy

As mentioned in the discussion of therapy for apraxia of speech, the fundamental principles that underlie therapy for the motor speech disorders (Darley, Aronson, & Brown, 1975, pp. 270–271) are applicable here.

Although various types of dysarthria have been delineated, therapy can be geared to the kind of speech problem rather than the type of dysarthria. There are some procedures that can be instituted prior to the onset of specific forms of therapy. Rosenbek and LaPointe (1978, pp. 276–286) indicate that speech performance is influenced by a structural and neuromuscular background, consisting of posture, muscle tone, and strength. Speech treatment can begin with attempts to modify this background, if such modification will improve speech or enhance the possibility for the success of techniques aimed specifically at the speech signal. They present in full detail the modification procedures (some of which are described below) for posture, muscle tone, and strength for general purposes and specifically for respiration, phonation, resonation, and articulation.

Netsell and Daniel (1979) suggest a physiologic approach to rehabilitation, which emphasizes the muscles and structure of respiration, the larynx, the velum and velopharyngeal area, the tongue blade, the tongue tip, the lips, and the mandible. This approach focuses on a component-by-component analysis of the peripheral speech mechanism in which the selection and sequencing of treatment follow directly from the physiologic nature and severity of involvement in each component. Recently, LaPointe (1982, pp. 370–400) and Rosenbek and LaPointe (1982) have advocated the physiologic approach in treating dysarthric patients.

Therapy for dysarthria can also be geared to the type of dysarthria rather than the kind of speech problem. In a recent book edited by Perkins (1984), a number of speech pathologists offer their own specific techniques in treating the dysarthric patient according to type. Included are treatment methods for flaccid dysarthria (Linebaugh, 1984b), spastic dysarthria (Aten, 1984), ataxic dysarthria (Murry, 1984), hypokinetic dysarthria (Berry, 1984), hyperkinetic dysarthria (Beukelman, 1984a), and mixed dysarthria (Beukelman, 1984b).

For problems in articulation, tongue depressors, mirrors, and counterresistant (strengthening) techniques can be used. Martin (1978) and Rosenbek and LaPointe (1978, pp. 284–286) have outlined lip exercises for strengthening the lip seal, for pursing, for lip elevation and closure, for lip depression and closure, and for lip retraction. Tongue strengthening exercises involve range of movement as well as tongue tip, lateral tongue, and posterior tongue movements. Dworkin (1980) suggests a program of isotonic or isometric tongue exercises prior to or in conjunction with phonetic training. Boone (1983, pp. 116–118) proposes additional techniques for altering tongue position. Chiefly for hypokinetic dysarthria, Berry (1984, pp. 91–99) recommends exaggerated chewing and slow and exaggerated alternate motion rate tasks to achieve maximal range of motion in articulation.

Netsell and Cleeland (1973) have proposed biofeedback from muscle activity as a way of reducing lip hypertonia. In later reports, Netsell (1978) and Netsell and Daniel (1979) have advocated the combined use of strengthening exercises (biting a block, pushing down on a depressor, etc.), biofeedback, a palatal lift, and instrumentation as aids to therapy for dysarthria. Although Darley, Aronson, and Brown (1975, pp. 272–274) question the value of techniques for strengthening the muscles, they do advocate slowing the rate of speech, a syllable-by-syllable attack (e.g., *af-ter-sup-per, when-ev-er-pos-si-ible*, etc.), and consonant exaggeration (e.g., ***important***, ***because***, etc.) as a means of increasing intelligibility in articulation. Primarily for hypokinetic dysarthria and often instead of traditional articulation therapy, Berry (1984, pp. 91–99) advocates slow rate control for producing intelligibility. It must be noted that strengthening exercises are contraindicated for conditions such as myasthenia gravis, where such exercises would produce a further weakening of the musculature (Darley, Aronson, & Brown, 1975, pp. 125–126; Rosenbek & LaPointe, 1978, p. 263).

Therapy that focuses on phoneme production begins with auditory training. This requires the use of the patient's auditory modality to first identify and name the erroneous sound. Subsequently, the patient learns to discriminate the stimulus sound from other sounds in simple and then more complex contexts. Boone (1983, pp. 135–139) offers additional techniques for ear training.

The phonetic placement method of describing the correct manner and place of articulation and the correct voiced and voiceless components of target phonemes production uses both visual and verbal instruction. The motokinesthetic approach, which is the manual manipulation of the articulators to produce the correct sound, can also be employed. This approach should be used with some caution since a study by Creech, Wertz, and Rosenbek (1973) has shown dysarthrics to be somewhat deficient in stereognostic abilities. Hartman, Day, and Pecora (1979) report using the phonetic placement and motokinesthetic approach along with Amerind signing with a dysarthric patient.

Since hypernasality is caused by insufficient movement of the velum, one intervention approach involves strengthening the muscles of the soft palate. Yawning and panting exercises can be used in conjunction with pushing techniques (Froeschels, Kastein, & Weiss, 1955). Pushing exercises require the patient to push with both arms and hands down upon a table top, upward under a table, hand against hand, or in parallel downward motion against the air.

Exercises using the back of the tongue (/kah/, /kay/, /kee/ and /gah/, /gay/, /gee/, etc.) can also be employed in strengthening the muscles of the soft palate. Here, the production of linguavelar consonants provides the stimulation to the soft palate. Another technique for reducing hypernasality involves directing the air stream through the oral cavity (Cole, 1972, pp. 250–258; Shelton, Hahn, & Morris, 1968, pp. 253–257). Straws, bubble pipes, oral-nasal cardboard platforms, Ping-Pong balls, horns, whistles, musical instruments, pinwheels, candles, balloons, feathers, and paper have all been used to refocus the direction of the air stream. Both the techniques of strengthening the muscles and of directing the air stream should be instituted with some caution since some studies (Baker & Sokoloff, 1951; Powers & Starr, 1974) have shown that these procedures may have little or no value in reducing hypernasality.

Tongue exercises (rotation, in and out) and lip exercises (pursing, puckering, retracting, biting down or up) are used to achieve flexibility. And, since a raised mandible and retracted tongue tend to isolate the oral cavity, thereby increasing the hypernasality, tongue and lip exercises are also used to prevent such movement. Appropriate exercises will hopefully open up the oral cavity as a resonator and combat the patient's attempts to retract the tongue or raise the mandible in an effort to reduce hypernasality. Boone (1983, pp. 118–123) outlines the use of biofeedback devices for cases of hypernasality.

The problem of strain-strangled voice is due to overadduction of the vocal cords. Therefore, the major thrust of therapy is aimed at attaining easy onset of phonation. One successful approach is the yawn-sigh technique, in which the patient is taught to produce phonation in an easy, relaxed yawn. The rationale for this technique is that yawning opens up the entire vocal tract, thereby cutting down on hyperadduction of the vocal cords. Another approach is to teach the patient to initiate phonation with the phoneme /h/, since this phoneme is produced with the vocal cords abducted and since it can eventually be employed to initiate the production of words and phrases.

Relaxation exercises centered around the head and neck area can also be used. Recently Rubow, Rosenbek, Collins, and Celesia (1984) reported using EMG biofeedback as a method for producing relaxation in successfully reducing the strain-strangled quality in a patient with hemifacial spasm and dysarthria.

Nemec and Cohen (1984) reported that EMG biofeedback was an effective treatment technique in a case of hypertonic spastic dysarthria.

Chewing exercises, which are based on the concept of eating, can be used for attaining relaxation and proper muscular tonus in the vocal tract. In a graduated series of steps patients are taught exaggerated chewing movements without and with phonation. Using these movements, the patient progresses from single-word phonation to conversational speech. Eventually the exaggerated movements are reduced to a point where the patient can chew mentally. Chewing exercises are described in detail by their originator, Froeschels (1952), and by Boone (1983, pp. 129–133).

Chiefly for spastic dysarthria, Aten (1984, pp. 69–77) suggests that all movements should be relaxed and slow to avoid triggering the spastic contractions and to retreat to a relaxed baseline whenever spasticity occurs. To reduce hyperadduction of the vocal cords, the clinician should start off with a relaxed, breathy sigh of short duration, proceed to short words beginning with /h/, then to open-mouth vowels, and then to a nasal consonant or continuant. Plosives and affricates are avoided because of the excessive pressure and musculature movement involved. Murry (1984, pp. 79–89) suggests the use of nasals and liquids to help "defuse" the explosive (strain-strangled) phonatory characteristics of Friedreich's ataxia. Additional exercises for easy phonation and relaxation are described by Boone (1983, pp. 141–143, 170–174).

The problem of breathiness results from insufficient glottal closure. Therefore, the main approach to therapy involves an attempt to close the glottis during phonation. For example, the previously described pushing exercises can be used to effect closure. Another approach based upon the pushing technique is the glottal attack using a phoneme. In this instance, the patient is taught to start hard contact phonation with a vowel or diphthong (/ah/, /ay/, /ee/, /aw/, /oh/, /oo/). This manner of initiating phonation is then applied to the production of words, phrases, and sentences. In cases of unilateral vocal-fold paralysis, Teflon and silicon injections (Darley, Aronson, & Brown, 1975, p. 277; Hammarberg, Fritzell, & Schiratzki, 1984) have been used to bolster or increase the size of the paralyzed cord. When the paralyzed cord is brought closer to the midline, better vocal-fold vibration is frequently possible.

Frequently, impairments in prosody can be alleviated by varying the patient's pitch and loudness. Exercises can be employed that help the patient discriminate auditorily while directing the pitch higher and lower. This therapy can begin with utterance of simple notes of the scale, then expand the vocalization to individual words and then to phrases. Loudness can be varied through the use of breathing exercises. Specifically, the patient is taught to be aware of the breathing cycle and then to control the exhalation phase during phonation. For example, the patient may initially be told to say "one, two" on one exhalation. Once this easy task is accomplished, the patient progresses to "three" and so on until he has both the phonation and exhalation required for the procedure under control. From there, he can vary the loudness of his voice commensurate with the degree of his breath control.

Another approach for prosody problems can be the use of phrasing through oral reading. Up and down arrows, pause marks, and metronomes can help with this approach. Both the "loudness" and "oral reading" approaches also place a strong emphasis on auditory training. Gradually these approaches can be introduced into spontaneous speech. Rubow (1984, pp. 207–230) found that rehabilitation based on visual biofeedback was superior to auditory training in achieving respiratory control in dysarthric subjects. Primarily for ataxic dysarthria, Murry (1984, pp. 75–89) notes that prosody problems are worked on by proper phrasing, slow rate, and loudness control. They all seem to work together. Boone (1983, pp. 164–165) offers additional suggestions for prosody improvement.

Hanson and Metler (1980; 1983, pp. 231–251) recently described how a delayed auditory feedback device was used to reduce speech rate and speech intelligibility in dysarthric speakers. Berry and Goshorn (1983, pp. 253–265), Caligiuri and Murry (1983, pp. 267–282), and Yorkston and Beukelman (1981c) reported using an oscilloscope as feedback for achieving rate control and intelligible speech with dysarthric patients. Murry (1983, pp. 69–83) has found that prosodic features in spastic, ataxic, and hypokinetic dysarthrics are different from those of normal subjects. Barnes (1983, pp. 57–68) reviews prosodic abnormalities in dysarthric speakers.

For loudness impairment, the breathing approaches described previously can be used to control loudness. The patient can also be helped to control intermittent loudness and inaudibility by being taught to slow down the rate of speech and produce a syllable-by-syllable mode of talking. Auditory training is essential to the development of self-monitoring skills for loudness levels. Since the respiratory process supplies the energy or force for speech, any impairment in this process should be properly evaluated and modified. Particularly for ataxic dysarthria, Murry (1984, pp. 79–89) suggests that loudness is rarely worked on alone. Proper phrasing and breathing and multisyllabic words are used to control loudness. Rosenbek and LaPointe (1978, pp. 286–290) review the instrumentation (biofeedback devices such as water manometers, air pressure transducers, etc.) and speech methods (postural adjustments, muscle strengthening, controlled exhalation, etc.) used in the diagnosis and treatment of respiratory problems. Recently McNamara (1983, pp. 191–201) noted the successful use of a biofeedback instrument with visual feedback to improve vocal loudness in a dysarthric patient.

For the severely dysarthric speaker, Calculator and Dollaghan (1982), Calculator and Luchko (1983), and McDonald and Schultz (1973) have reviewed the various types of communication boards that can be used. They include picture boards, word and phrase boards, and boards for sentence construction. Although some of these communication boards are geared for severe motorically involved children, they can be adapted for use with dysarthric adults. Beukelman and Yorkston (1977) have described a communication system that improves intelligibility in the severely dysarthric speaker with an intact language system. These authors suggest that letters, numbers, and directions such as "repeat," "start again," "end of word," and "end of sentence" be mounted on a board and that patients be taught to point to the first letter of each word as they speak. Fristoe and Lloyd (1980) suggest an expressive sign lexicon based on those used with retarded and autistic persons. Several electronic units (Goodenough-Trepagnier & Prather, 1981; Steadman, Ferris, & Rhodine, 1980), a portable tape typewriter (Beukelman et al., 1981), and microcomputer-based augmentative communication systems (Linebaugh, Baird, Baird, & Armour, 1983, pp. 295–303) have been used successfully with severely involved neuromotor patients.

In cases of severe velopharyngeal competency, a palatal lift may be used to aid in producing closure of that area. This prosthesis is attached to the teeth and is made in the shape of a bulb obturator with a hard plastic shelf attached to the posterior section of the palatal portion. This shelf projects posteriorly under the soft palate and maintains the palate in an elevated position (Hardy, Netsell, Schweiger, & Morris, 1969). With the use of a palatal lift, success has been noted in reducing hypernasality and nasal emission and in increasing the overall intelligibility of speech in dysarthic children (Hardy, Netshell, Schweiger, & Morris, 1969; Netsell, 1969; Kent & Netsell, 1978), in developmentally delayed children (Shaughnessy, Netsell, & Farrage, 1983, pp. 217–230), and in dysarthric adults (Aten, McDonald, Simpson, & Gutierez, 1984, pp. 231–241; Gibbons & Bloomer, 1958; Gonzalez & Aronson, 1970; Netshell, 1978; Netshell & Daniel, 1979). Additional reviews of instrumentation and speech methods used in the treatment of dysarthria can be found in Boone (1983), Berry and Sanders (1983, pp. 203–216), Beukelman (1984b, pp. 105–113), Darley, Aronson, and Brown (1975, pp. 270–278), Halpern (1981, pp. 347–360), Johns and Salyer (1978, pp. 311–331), Linebaugh (1984b, pp. 59–67), Rosenbek and LaPointe (1978, pp. 251–310), Schuell, Jenkins, and Jimenez-Pabon (1964, pp. 362–365), and Wolfe, Ratusnik, and Penn (1981). Reviews of nonspeech communication can be found in Silverman (1984, pp. 115–121), Yoder and Kraat (1983, pp. 27–51), and Yorkston and Dowden (1984, pp. 283–312).

In summary, dysarthria can be viewed as a motoric problem that involves the speech and/or vocal musculature. It exists neither on a linguistic level, as does aphasia, nor on a programming or transmissive level, as apraxia of speech. These patients are consistent in their errors, have no difficulty in starting speech, lack the ability to give a correct production after a number of faulty attempts, and do not improve when speaking automatically or volitionally. They are frustrated when in error; their syntactic and semantic qualities should be intact; their responses are relevant to the situation; and their memory, thinking, and abstracting abilities should not be impaired. Dysarthria is a motor problem that can affect articulation, voice, breathing, resonance, and prosody.

References

Abbs, J., Hunker, C., & Barlow, S. (1983). Differential speech motor subsystems impairments with suprabulbar lesions: Neurophysiological framework and supporting data. In W. Berry (Ed.), *Clinical dysarthria* (pp. 21–56). San Diego: College Hill Press.

Alpert, M. (1981). Speech and disturbance of affect. In J. Darby (Ed.), *Speech evaluation in psychiatry* (pp. 359–367). New York: Grune & Stratton.

Ansel, B., McNeil, M., Hunker, C., & Bliss, D. (1983). The frequency of verbal and acoustic adjustments used by cerebral palsied dysarthric adults when faced with communicative failure. In W. Berry (Ed.), *Clinical dysarthria* (pp. 85–106). San Diego: College Hill Press.

Appell, J., Kertesz, A., & Fisman, M. (1982). A study of language functioning in Alzheimer's patients. *Brain and Language, 17,* 73–91.

Aronson, A. (1980). *Clinical voice disorders.* New York: Thieme-Stratton.

Aten, J. (1984). Treatment of spastic dysarthria. In W. Perkins (Ed.), *Dysarthria and apraxia* (pp. 69–77). New York: Thieme-Stratton.

Aten, J., Caligiuri, M., & Holland, A. (1982). The efficacy of functional communication therapy for chronic aphasic patients. *Journal of Speech and Hearing Disorders, 47,* 93–96.

Aten, J., Johns, D., & Darley, F. (1971). Auditory perception of sequenced words in apraxia of speech. *Journal of Speech and Hearing Research, 14,* 131–143.

Aten, J., McDonald, A., Simpson, M., & Gutierez, R. (1984). Efficacy of modified palatal lifts for improving resonance. In M. McNeil, J. Rosenbek, & A. Aronson (Eds.), *The dysarthrias: Physiology, acoustics, perceptions, management* (pp. 231–241). San Diego: College Hill Press.

Baker, E., & Sokoloff, M. (1951). Therapy for speech deficiencies resulting from acute bulbar poliomyelitis infection. *Journal of Speech and Hearing Disorders, 16,* 337–339.

Barlow, S., & Abbs, J. (1983). Force transducers for the evaluation of labial, lingual, and mandibular motor impairments. *Journal of Speech and Hearing Research, 26,* 616–621.

Barlow, S., Cole, K., & Abbs, J. (1983). A new head-mounted lip-jaw movement transduction system for the study of motor speech disorders. *Journal of Speech and Hearing Research, 26,* 283–288.

Barnes, G. (1983). Suprasegmental and prosodic considerations in motor speech disorders. In W. Berry (Ed.), *Clinical dysarthria* (pp. 57–68). San Diego: College Hill Press.

Basso, A., Capitani, E., & Vignolo, L. A. (1979). Influence of rehabilitation on language skills in aphasic patients: A controlled study. *Archives of Neurology, 36,* 190–196.

Bayles, K. (1982). Language function in senile dementia. *Brain and Language, 16,* 265–280.

Bayles, K. (1984). Language and dementia. In A. Holland (Ed.), *Language disorders in adults* (pp. 209–244). San Diego: College Hill Press.

Bayles, K., & Boone, D. (1982). The potential of language tasks for identifying senile dementia. *Journal of Speech and Hearing Disorders, 47*, 210–217.

Bayles, K., & Tomoeda, C. (1983). Confrontation naming impairment in dementia. *Brain and Language, 19*, 98–114.

Bayles, K., Tomoeda, C., & Caffrey, J. (1982). Language and dementia-producing diseases. *Communicative Disorders, 7*, 131–146.

Bemporad, J., & Pinsker, H. (1974). Schizophrenia: The manifest symptomatology. In S. Arieti & E. Brody (Eds.), *American handbook of psychiatry* (Vol. 3, pp. 524–550). New York: Basic Books.

Benson, D. F. (1973). Psychiatric aspects of aphasia. *British Journal of Psychiatry, 123*, 555–556.

Benson, D. F. (1979). *Aphasia, alexia, agraphia*. New York: Churchill, Livingstone.

Bentin, S., Silverberg, R., & Gordon, H. (1981). Asymmetrical cognitive deterioration in demented and Parkinson patients. *Cortex, 17*, 533–544.

Benton, A., & Hamsher, K. (1978). *Multilingual aphasia examination*. Iowa City: Benton Laboratory of Neuropsychology.

Berndt, R., & Caramazza, A. (1981). Syntactic aspects of aphasia. In M. Sarno (Ed.), *Acquired aphasia* (pp. 157–182). New York: Academic Press.

Berry, W. (1984). Treatment of hypokinetic dysarthria. In W. Perkins (Ed.), *Dysarthria and apraxia* (pp. 91–99). New York: Thieme-Stratton.

Berry, W., Darley, F., Aronson, A., & Goldstein, N. (1974). Dysarthria in Wilson's disease. *Journal of Speech and Hearing Research, 17*, 169–183.

Berry, W., & Goshorn, E. (1983). Immediate visual feedback in the treatment of ataxic dysarthria: A case study. In W. Berry (Ed.), *Clinical dysarthria* (pp. 253–265). San Diego: College Hill Press.

Berry, W., & Sanders, S. (1983). Environmental education: The universal management approach for adults with dysarthria. In W. Berry (Ed.), *Clinical dysarthria* (pp. 203–216). San Diego: College Hill Press.

Beukelman, D. (1984a). Treatment of hyperkinetic dysarthria. In W. Perkins (Ed.), *Dysarthria and apraxia* (pp. 101–103). New York: Thieme-Stratton.

Beukelman, D. (1984b). Treatment of mixed dysarthria. In W. Perkins (Ed.), *Dysarthria and apraxia* (pp. 105–113). New York: Thieme-Stratton.

Beukelman, D., & Yorkston, K. (1977). A communication system for the severely dysarthric speaker with an intact language system. *Journal of Speech and Hearing Disorders, 42*, 265–270.

Beukelman, D., & Yorkston, K. (1979). The relationship between information transfer and speech intelligibility of dysarthric speakers. *Journal of Communication Disorders, 12*, 189–196.

Beukelman, D., & Yorkston, K. (1980a). Influence of passage familiarity on intelligibility estimates of dysarthric speech. *Journal of Communication Disorders, 13*, 33–41.

Beukelman, D., & Yorkston, K. (1980b). Nonvocal communication: Performance evaluation. *Archives of Physical Medicine and Rehabilitation, 61*, 273–275.

Beukelman, D., Yorkston, K., Gorhoff, S., Mitsuda, P., & Kenyon, V. (1981). Canon communicator use by adults: A retrospective study. *Journal of Speech and Hearing Disorders, 46*, 374–378.

Beukelman, D., Yorkston, K., & Waugh, P. (1980). Communication in severe aphasia: Effectiveness of three instruction modalities. *Archives of Physical Medicine and Rehabilitation, 61*, 248–252.

Blumstein, S. (1981). Phonological aspects of aphasia. In M. Sarno (Ed.), *Acquired aphasia* (pp. 129–155). New York: Academic Press.

Boone, D. (1983). *The voice and voice therapy*. Englewood Cliffs, NJ: Prentice-Hall.

Borkowski, J., Benton, A., & Spreen, O. (1967). Word fluency and brain damage. *Neuropsychologia, 5*, 135–140.

Brookshire, R. (1967). Speech pathology and the experimental analysis of behavior. *Journal of Speech and Hearing Disorders, 32*, 215–227.

Brookshire, R. (1978). Auditory comprehension in aphasia. In D. Johns (Ed.), *Clinical management of neurogenic disorders* (pp. 103–128). Boston: Little, Brown.

Brookshire, R. (1983). Subject description and generality of results in experiments with aphasic adults. *Journal of Speech and Hearing Disorders, 48*, 342–346.

Brosin, H. (1967). Acute and chronic brain syndromes. In A. Friedman & H. Kaplan (Eds.), *Comprehensive textbook of psychiatry* (pp. 708–711). Baltimore: Williams & Wilkins.

Buckingham, H. (1979). Explanation in apraxia with consequences for the concept of apraxia of speech. *Brain and Language, 8*, 202–226.

Buckingham, H. (1981). Lexical and semantic aspects of aphasia. In M. Sarno (Ed.), *Acquired aphasia* (pp. 183–214). New York: Academic Press.

Burns, M., & Canter, G. (1977). Phonemic behavior of aphasic patients with posterior cerebral lesions. *Brain and Language, 4*, 492–507.

Calculator, S., & Dollaghan, C. (1982). The use of communication boards in a residential setting: An evaluation. *Journal of Speech and Hearing Disorders, 47*, 281–287.

Calculator, S., & Luchko, C. (1983). Evaluating the effectiveness of a communication board testing program. *Journal of Speech and Hearing Disorders, 48*, 185–191.

Caligiuri, M., & Murry, T. (1983). The use of visual feedback to enhance prosodic control in dysarthria. In W. Berry (Ed.), *Clinical dysarthria* (pp. 267–282). San Diego: College Hill Press.

Canter, G. (1967). Neuromotor pathologies of speech. *American Journal of Physical Medicine, 46*, 659–666.

Caramazza, A. (1984). The logic of neuropsychological research and the problem of patient classification in aphasia. *Brain and Language, 21*, 9–20.

Chaika, E. (1974). A linguist looks at schizophrenic language. *Brain and Language, 1*, 257–276.

Chaika, E. (1977). Schizophrenic speech, slips of the tongue, and jargon-aphasia: A reply to Fromkin and to Lecours and Venier-Clement. *Brain and Language, 4*, 464–475.

Chaika, E. (1982). A unified explanation for the diverse structural deviations reported for adult schizophrenics with disrupted speech. *Journal of Communication Disorders, 15*, 167–189.

Chapey, R. (1981a). The assessment of language disorders in adults. In R. Chapey (Ed.), *Language intervention strategies in adult aphasia* (pp. 31–84). Baltimore: Williams & Wilkins.

Chapey, R. (1981b). Divergent semantic intervention. In R. Chapey (Ed.), *Language intervention strategies in aphasia* (pp. 155–167). Baltimore: Williams & Wilkins.

Chapey, R. (1983). Language-based cognitive abilities in adult aphasia: Rationale for intervention. *Journal of Communication Disorders, 16*, 405–424.

Chapman, J. (1966). The early symptoms of schizophrenia. *British Journal of Psychiatry, 112*, 225–251.

Chedru, F., & Geschwind, N. (1972). Higher cortical functions in confusional states. *Cortex, 8*, 397–409.

Cohen, R., Engel, D., Kelter, S., List, G., & Stroehner, H. (1977). Validity of the Sklar aphasia scale. *Journal of Speech and Hearing Research, 20*, 146–154.

Cole, R. (1972). Direct muscle training for the improvement of velopharyngeal function. In K. Bzoch (Ed.), *Communicative disorders related to cleft palate* (pp. 250–256). Boston: Little, Brown.

Coleman, C., Cook, A., & Meyers, L. (1980). Assessing non-oral clients for assistive communication devices. *Journal of Speech and Hearing Disorders, 45*, 515–520.

Costello, J. (1977). Programmed instruction. *Journal of Speech and Hearing Disorders, 42*, 3–28.

Collins, M. (1983). Global aphasia: Knowledge in search of understanding. *Communicative Disorders, 8*, 125–137.

Collins, M. (1984). Integrating perceptual and instrumental procedures in dysarthria assessment. *Communicative Disorders, 9*, 159–170.

Collins, M., Rosenbek, J., & Wertz, R. (1983). Spectographic analysis of vowel and word duration in apraxia of speech. *Journal of Speech and Hearing Research, 26*, 224–230.

Creech, R., Wertz, R., & Rosenbek, J. (1973). Oral sensation and perception in dysarthric adults. *Perceptual and Motor Skills, 37*, 167–172.

Critchley, M. (1964). The neurology of psychotic speech. *British Journal of Psychiatry, 110*, 353–364.

Critchley, M. (1970). *Aphasiology and other aspects of language*. London: Edward Arnold.

Cummings, J., & Benson, D. F. (1983). *Dementia: A clinical approach*. Boston: Butterworths.

Dabul, B. (1979). *Apraxia battery for adults*. Tigard, OR: C. C. Publications.

Dabul, B., & Bollier, B. (1976). Therapeutic approaches to apraxia. *Journal of Speech and Hearing Disorders, 41*, 268–276.

Damasio, A. (1981). The nature of aphasia: Signs and syndromes. In M. Sarno (Ed.), *Acquired aphasia*, (pp. 51–66). New York: Academic Press.

Darby, J. (1981). Speech and voice studies in psychiatric populations. In J. Darby (Ed.), *Speech evaluation in psychiatry* (pp. 253–284). New York: Grune & Stratton.

Darby, J., Simmons, N., & Berger, P. (1984). Speech and voice parameters of depression: A pilot study. *Journal of Communication Disorders, 17*, 75–85.

Darley, F. (1964). *Diagnosis and appraisal of communicative disorders*. Englewood Cliffs, NJ: Prentice-Hall.

Darley, F. (1969). *Nomenclature of expressive speech disturbances resulting from lesions of Broca's area: 108 years of proliferation and confusion.* Paper presented at the meeting of the Academy of Aphasia, Boston.

Darley, F. (1972). The efficacy of language rehabilitation in aphasia. *Journal of Speech and Hearing Disorders, 37,* 3–21.

Darley, F. (Ed.). (1979). *Evaluation of appraisal techniques in speech and language pathology*. Reading, MA: Addison-Wesley.

Darley, F. (1982). *Aphasia*. Philadelphia: Saunders.

Darley, F., Aronson, A., & Brown, J. (1969a). Differential diagnostic patterns of dysarthria. *Journal of Speech and Hearing Research, 12,* 246–269.

Darley, F., Aronson, A., & Brown, J. (1969b). Clusters of deviant speech dimensions in the dysarthrias. *Journal of Speech and Hearing Research, 12,* 462–496.

Darley, F., Aronson, A., & Brown, J. (1975). *Motor speech disorders.* Philadelphia: Saunders.

Darley, F., Brown, J., & Goldstein, N. (1972). Dysarthria in multiple sclerosis. *Journal of Speech and Hearing Research, 15,* 229–245.

Darley, F., & Spriestersbach, D. (1978). *Diagnostic methods in speech pathology.* New York: Harper & Row.

Davis, G. (1983). *A survey of adult aphasia.* Englewood Cliffs, NJ: Prentice-Hall.

Davis, G., & Wilcox, J. (1981). Incorporating parameters of natural conversation in aphasia treatment. In R. Chapey (Ed.), *Language intervention strategies in adult aphasia* (pp. 169–193). Baltimore: Williams & Wilkins.

Day, M., & Semrad, E. (1978). Schizophrenic reactions. In A. Nicholi (Ed.), *The Harvard guide to modern psychiatry* (pp. 191–241). Cambridge, MA: Harvard University Press.

Deal, J. (1974). Consistency and adaptation in apraxia of speech. *Journal of Communication Disorders, 7,* 135–140.

Deal, J., & Darley, F. (1972). The influence of linguistic and situational variables on phonemic accuracy in apraxia of speech. *Journal of Speech and Hearing Research, 15,* 639–653.

Deal, J., & Florance, C. (1978). Modification of the eight-step continuum for treatment of apraxia of speech in adults. *Journal of Speech and Hearing Disorders, 43,* 89–95.

Deal, J., Wertz, R., & Spring, C. (1981). Differentiating aphasia and the language of generalized intellectual impairment. In R. Brookshire (Ed.), *Clinical aphasiology: Proceedings of the conference* (pp. 166–173). Minneapolis: BRK Publishers.

DeFeo, A., & Schaefer, C. (1983). Bilateral facial paralysis in a preschool child: Oral-facial and articulatory characteristics (a case study). In W. Berry (Ed.), *Clinical dysarthria* (pp. 165–186). San Diego: College Hill Press.

DeRenzi, E., & Ferrari, C. (1978). The reporter's test: A sensitive test to detect expressive disturbances in aphasics. *Cortex, 14,* 279–293.

DeRenzi, E., Peizcuro, A., & Vignolo, L.(1966). Oral apraxia and aphasia. Cortex, *2,* 50–73.

DeRenzi, E., & Vignolo, L. (1962). The token test: A sensitive test to detect receptive disturbances in aphasics. *Brain, 85*, 665–678.

Deutsch, S. (1981). Oral form identification as a measure of cortical sensory dysfunction in apraxia of speech and aphasia. *Journal of Communication Disorders, 14*, 65–73.

Deutsch, S. (1984). Predictions of site of lesions from speech apraxic error patterns. In J. Rosenbek, M. McNeil, & A. Aronson (Eds.), *Apraxia of speech: Physiology, acoustics, linguistics, management* (pp. 113–134). San Diego: College Hill Press.

DiCarlo, L. (1980). Language recovery in aphasia: Effect of systematic filmed programmed instruction. *Archives of Physical Medicine and Rehabilitation, 61*, 41–44.

DiSimoni, F. (1981). Therapies which utilize alternate or augmentative communication systems. In R. Chapey (Ed.), *Language intervention strategies in adult aphasia* (pp. 329–346). Baltimore: Williams & Wilkins.

DiSimoni, F., & Darley, F. (1977). Effect on phoneme duration control of three utterance-length conditions in an apractic patient. *Journal of Speech and Hearing Disorders, 42*, 257–264.

DiSimoni, F., Darley, F., & Aronson, A. (1977). Patterns of dysfunction in schizophrenic patients on an aphasia test battery. *Journal of Speech and Hearing Disorders, 42*, 498–513.

Drummond, S. (1984). *Characterization of irrelevant speech: A case study*. Unpublished manuscript. (Available from University of Arkansas for Medical Sciences, 4301 West Markham, Little Rock, AR 72205)

Duffy, J. (1981). Schuell's stimulation approach to rehabilitation. In R. Chapey (Ed.), *Language intervention strategies in adult aphasia* (pp. 105–139). Baltimore: Williams & Wilkins.

Duffy, J., & Garole, C. (1984). Apraxic speakers' vowel duration in consonant-vowel-consonant syllables. In J. Rosenbek, M. McNeil, & A. Aronson (Eds.), *Apraxia of speech: Physiology, acoustics, linguistics, management* (pp. 167–196). San Diego: College Hill Press.

Dunlop, J., & Marquardt, T. (1977). Linguistic and articulatory aspects of single word production in apraxia of speech. *Cortex, 13*, 17–29.

Dworkin, J. (1980). Tongue strength measurement in patients with amyotrophic lateral sclerosis: Qualitative vs. quantitative procedures. *Archives of Physical Medicine and Rehabilitation, 61*, 422–424.

Dworkin, J., Aronson, A., & Mulder, D. (1980). Tongue force in normals and in dysarthric patients with amyotrophic lateral sclerosis. *Journal of Speech and Hearing Research, 23*, 828–837.

Eisenson, J. (1949). Prognostic factors related to language rehabilitation in aphasic patients. *Journal of Speech and Hearing Disorders, 14*, 262–264.

Eisenson, J. (1954). *Examining for aphasia*. New York: Psychological Corporation.

Eisenson, J. (1981). Issues, prognosis, and problems in the rehabilitation of language disorders in adults. In R. Chapey (Ed.), *Language intervention strategies in adult aphasia* (pp. 85–101). Baltimore: Williams & Wilkins.

Eisenson, J. (1984). *Adult aphasia*. Englewood Cliffs, NJ: Prentice-Hall.

Emerick, L., & Hatten, J. (1974). *Diagnosis and evaluation in speech pathology.* Englewood Cliffs, NJ: Prentice-Hall.

Enderby, P. (1983a). The standardized measurement of dysarthria is possible. In W. Berry (Ed.), *Clinical dysarthria* (pp. 109–119). San Diego: College Hill Press.

Enderby, P. (1983b). *Frenchay dysarthria assessment*. San Diego: College Hill Press.

Estabrooks, N. (1981). *Helm elicited language program for syntax stimulation*. Austin, TX: Exceptional Resources.

Fish, F. (1957). The classification of schizophrenia: The views of Kleist and his co-workers. *Journal of Mental Science, 103,* 443–463.

Fitch, J., & Cross, S. (1983). Telecomputer treatment for aphasia. *Journal of Speech and Hearing Disorders, 48,* 335–336.

Fitch-West, J. (1984). Aphasia rehabilitation. In S. Dickson (Ed.), *Communication disorders: Remedial principles and practices* (pp. 378–445). Glenview, IL: Scott-Foresman.

Fristoe, M., & Lloyd, L. (1980). Planning an initial expressive sign lexicon for persons with severe communication impairment. *Journal of Speech and Hearing Disorders, 45,* 170–180.

Froeschels, E. (1943). A contribution to the pathology and therapy of dysarthria due to certain cerebral lesions. *Journal of Speech and Hearing Disorders, 8,* 301–321.

Froeschels, E. (1952). Chewing method as therapy. *Archives of Otolaryngology, 56,* 427–434.

Froeschels, E., Kastein, S., & Weiss, D. (1955). A method of therapy for paralytic conditions of the mechanisms of phonation, respiration, and glutination. *Journal of Speech and Hearing Disorders, 20,* 365–370.

Gardner, H., Zurif, E., Berry, T., & Baker, E. (1976). Visual communication in aphasia. *Neuropsychologia, 14,* 275–292.

Gerson, S., Benson, D. F., & Frazier, S. (1977). Diagnosis: Schizophrenia versus posterior aphasia. *American Journal of Psychiatry, 134,* 966–969.

Geschwind, N. (1967). The varieties of naming errors. *Cortex, 3,* 97–112.

Gewirth, L., Shindler, A., & Hier, D. (1984). Altered patterns of word associations in dementia and aphasia. *Brain and Language, 21,* 307–317.

Gibbons, P., & Bloomer, H. (1958). A supportive-type prosthetic speech aid. *Journal of Prosthetic Dentistry, 8,* 362–369.

Goldfarb, R. (1981). Operant conditioning and programmed instruction in aphasia rehabilitation. In R. Chapey (Ed.), *Language intervention strategies in adult aphasia* (pp. 249–263). Baltimore: Williams & Wilkins.

Golper, L., Nutt, J., Rau, M., & Coleman, R. (1983). Focalcranial dystonia. *Journal of Speech and Hearing Disorders, 48,* 128–134.

Gonzalez, J., & Aronson, A. (1970). Palatal lift prosthesis for treatment of anatomic and neurologic palatopharyngeal insufficiency. *Cleft Palate Journal, 7,* 91–104.

Goodglass, H., & Kaplan, E. (1983). *The assessment of aphasia and related disorders* (2nd ed). Philadelphia: Lea & Febiger.

Goodenough-Trepagnier, C., & Prather, P. (1981). Communication systems for the non-vocal based on frequent phoneme sequences. *Journal of Speech and Hearing Research, 24,* 322–329.

Grewel, F. (1957). Classification of dysarthrias. *Acta Psychiatrica Scand., 32*, 325–337.

Groher, M. (1977). Language and memory disorders following closed head trauma. *Journal of Speech and Hearing Research, 20*, 212–223.

Grunwell, P., & Huskins, S. (1979). Intelligibility in acquired dysarthria – a neurophonetic approach: Three case studies. *Journal of Communication Disorders, 12*, 9–22.

Guilford, A., Scheuerle, J., & Shirek, P. (1982). Manual communication skills in aphasia. *Archives of Physical Medicine and Rehabilitation, 63*, 601–604.

Hagen, C. (1984). Language disorders in head trauma. In A. Holland (Ed.), *Language disorders in adults* (pp. 245–281). San Diego: College Hill Press.

Halpern, H. (1978). Evaluation of linguistic disorders in adults. In S. Singh & J. Lynch (Eds.), *Diagnostic procedures in hearing, speech, and language* (pp. 379–409). Austin, TX: PRO-ED.

Halpern, H. (1980). The differential diagnosis of speech and language impairment in the adult neuropsychiatric patient. In L. Bradford & T. Wertz (Eds.), *Communicative Disorders: An Audio Journal for Continuing Education, 5*, (4).

Halpern, H. (1981). Therapy for agnosia, apraxia, and dysarthria. In R. Chapey (Ed.), *Language intervention strategies in adult aphasia* (pp. 347–360). Baltimore: Williams & Wilkins.

Halpern, H., Darley, F., & Brown, J. (1973). Differential language and neurologic characteristics in cerebral involvement. *Journal of Speech and Hearing Disorders, 38*, 162–173.

Halpern, H., & McCartin-Clark, M. (1984). Differential language characteristics in adult aphasic and schizophrenic subjects. *Journal of Communication Disorders, 17*, 289–307.

Hammarberg, B., Fritzell, B., & Schiratzki, H. (1984). Teflon injection in 16 patients with paralytic dysphonia: Perceptual and acoustic evaluations. *Journal of Speech and Hearing Disorders, 49*, 78–82.

Hanson, W., & Metler, E. (1980). DAF as instrumental treatment for dysarthria in progressive supranuclear palsy: A case report. *Journal of Speech and Hearing Disorders, 45*, 268–276.

Hanson, W., & Metler, E. (1983). DAF speech-rate modification in Parkinson's disease: A report of two cases. In W. Berry (Ed.), *Clinical dysarthria* (pp. 231–251). San Diego: College Hill Press.

Hardison, D., Marquardt, T., & Peterson, H. (1977). Effects of selected linguistic variables on apraxia of speech. *Journal of Speech and Hearing Research, 20*, 334–343.

Hardy, J., Netsell, R., Schweiger, J., & Morris, H. (1969). Management of velopharyngeal dysfunction in cerebral palsy. *Journal of Speech and Hearing Disorders, 34*, 123–136.

Hartman, D., Day, M., & Pecora, R. (1979). Treatment of dysarthria: A case report. *Journal of Communication Disorders, 12*, 167–173.

Hecaen, H. (1972). *Introduction à la neuropsychologie*. Paris: Larousse.

Helm, N., & Benson, F. (1978). *Visual action therapy for global aphasia*. Paper presented at the meeting of the Academy of Aphasia, Chicago.

Helm-Estabrooks, N. (1983). Language intervention for adults: Environmental considerations. In J. Miller, D. Yoder, & R. Schiefelbusch (Eds.), *Contemporary issues in language intervation* (Report No. 12, pp. 229–238). Rockville, MD: American Speech-Language-Hearing Association.

Helm-Estabrooks, N. (1984). Severe aphasia. In A. Holland (Ed.), *Language disorders in adults* (pp. 159–176). San Diego: College Hill Press.

Helm-Estabrooks, N., Fitzpatrick, P., & Barresi, B. (1982). Visual action therapy for global aphasia. *Journal of Speech and Hearing Disorders, 47*, 385–389.

Herbert, R., & Waltensperger, K. (1980). Schizophrenia: Case study of a paranoid schizophrenic's language. *Applied Psycholinguistics, 1*, 81–93.

Hilton, L., & Kraetschmer, K. (1983). International trends in aphasia rehabilitation. *Archives of Physical Medicine and Rehabilitation, 64*, 462–467.

Hirose, H., Kiritani, S., Ushijima, T., & Sawashima, M. (1978). Analysis of abnormal articulatory dynamics in two dysarthric patients. *Journal of Speech and Hearing Disorders, 43*, 96–105.

Hixon, T., Putnam, A., & Sharp, J. (1983). Speech production with flaccid paralysis of the rib cage, diaphragm, and abdomen. *Journal of Speech and Hearing Disorders, 48*, 315–327.

Hoffman, R., Kirstein, L., Stopek, S., & Cicchetti, D. (1982). Apprehending schizophrenic discourse: A structural analysis of the listener's task. *Brain and Language, 15*, 207–233.

Hoffman, R., & Sledge, W. (1984). A microgenetic model of paragrammatisms produced by a schizophrenic speaker. *Brain and Language, 21*, 147–173.

Hoit-Dalgaard, J., Murry, T., & Kopp, H. (1983). Voice onset time production and perception in apraxic subjects. *Brain and Language, 20*, 329–339.

Holland, A. (1970). Case studies in aphasia rehabilitation using programmed instructions. *Journal of Speech and Hearing Disorders, 35*, 377–390.

Holland, A. (1980). *Communicative abilities in daily living.* Austin, TX: PRO-ED.

Holland, A. (1982a). Observing functional communication of aphasic adults. *Journal of Speech and Hearing Disorders, 47*, 50–56.

Holland, A. (1982b). Aphasia in adults. In G. Shames & E. Wiig (Eds.), *Human communication disorders* (pp. 434–438). Columbus, OH: Merrill.

Holland, A. (1983). Language intervention in adults: What is it? In J. Miller, D. Yoder, & R. Schiefelbusch (Eds.), *Contemporary issues in language intervention* (Report No. 12, pp. 3–12). Rockville, MD: American Speech-Language-Hearing Association.

Hoops, H. (1980). Language disorders in adults. In R. Van Hattum (Ed.), *Communication disorders: An introduction* (pp. 337–375). New York: Macmillan.

Horner, J. (1984). Moderate aphasia. In A. Holland (Ed.), *Language disorders in adults* (pp. 133–157). San Diego: College Hill Press.

Horner, J., Heipman, A., Aker, C., Kanter, J., & Royall, J. (1982, Oct.). *Misnaming of Alzheimer's dementia compared to misnamings associated with left and right hemisphere stroke.* Paper presented at the meeting of the Academy of Aphasia, Lake Mohonk, NY.

Horsfall, G. (1972). *An investigation of selected language performance in adult schizophrenic subjects.* Unpublished doctoral dissertation, University of Florida.

Hunker, C., & Abbs, J. (1984). Physiological analysis of Parkinsonian tremors in the orofacial system. In M. McNeil, J. Rosenbek, & A. Aronson (Eds.), *The dysarthrias: Physiology, acoustics, perception, management* (pp. 69–100). San Diego: College Hill Press.

Itoh, M., & Sasanuma, S. (1984). Articulatory movements in apraxia of speech. In J. Rosenbek, M. McNeil, & A. Aronson (Eds.), *Apraxia of speech: Physiology, acoustics, linguistics, management* (pp. 135–165). San Diego: College Hill Press.

Itoh, M., Sasanuma, S., Hirose, H., Yoshioka, H., & Ushijima, T. (1980). Abnormal articulatory dynamics in a patient with apraxia of speech: X-ray microbeam observations. *Brain and Language, 11*, 66–75.

Itoh, M., Sasanuma, S., Tatsumi, I., Murakami, S., Fukusako, Y., & Suzuki, T. (1982). Voice onset time characteristics in apraxia of speech. *Brain and Language, 17*, 193–210.

Joanette, Y., & Dudley, J. (1980). Dysarthic symptomatology of Fredreich's ataxia. *Brain and Language, 10*, 39–50.

Johns, D., & Darley, F. (1970). Phonemic variability in apraxia of speech. *Journal of Speech and Hearing Research, 13*, 556–583.

Johns, D., & LaPointe, L. (1976). Neurogenic disorders of output processing: Apraxia of speech. In H. Whitaker & H. Whitaker (Eds.), *Studies in neurolinguistics I* (pp. 161–199). New York: Academic Press.

Johns, D., & Salyer, K. (1978). Surgical and prosthetic management of neurogenic speech disorders. In D. Johns (Ed.), *Clinical management of neurogenic communicative disorders* (pp. 311–331). Boston: Little, Brown.

Karanth, P. (1981). The disorders of language in aphasia and psychoses. *International Journal of Dravidian Linguistics, 10*, 336–343.

Kaszniak, A., Garron, D., & Fox, J. (1979). Differential effects of age and cerebral atrophy upon span of immediate recall and paired-associate learning in older patients suspected of dementia. *Cortex, 15*, 285–295.

Keenan, J., & Brassell, E. (1975). *Aphasia language performance scales.* Murfreesboro, TN: Pinnacle Press.

Keith, R., & Aronson, A. (1975). Singing as therapy for apraxia of speech and aphasia: Report of a case. *Brain and Language, 2*, 483.

Kelso, J., & Tuller, B. (1981). Toward a theory of apractic syndromes. *Brain and Language, 12*, 224–245.

Keller, E. (1984). Simplification and gesture reduction in phonological disorders of apraxia and aphasia. In J. Rosenbek, M. McNeil, & A. Aronson (Eds.), *Apraxia of speech: Physiology, acoustics, linguistics, management* (pp. 221–256). San Diego: College Hill Press.

Kent, R., & Netsell, R. (1975). A case study of an ataxic dysarthric: Cineradiographic and spectrographic observations. *Journal of Speech and Hearing Disorders, 40*, 115–133.

Kent, R., & Netsell, R. (1978). Articulatory abnormalities in athetoid cerebral palsy. *Journal of Speech and Hearing Disorders, 43*, 353–373.

Kent, R., Netsell, R., & Abbs, J. (1979). Acoustic characteristics of dysarthria associated with cerebellar disease. *Journal of Speech and Hearing Research, 22,* 627–648.

Kent, R., & Rosenbek, J. (1982). Prosodic disturbance and neurologic lesion. *Brain and Language, 15,* 259–291.

Kent, R., & Rosenbek, J. (1983). Acoustic patterns of apraxia of speech. *Journal of Speech and Hearing Research, 26,* 231–249.

Kertesz, A. (1979). *Aphasia and associated disorders: Taxonomy, localization, and recovery.* New York: Grune & Stratton.

Kertesz, A. (1984). Subcortical lesions and verbal apraxia. In J. Rosenbek, M. McNeil, & A. Aronson (Eds.), *Apraxia of speech: Physiology, acoustics, linguistics, management* (pp. 73–90). San Diego: College Hill Press.

Kertesz, A., & Poole, E. (1974). The aphasia quotient: The taxonomic approach to measurement of aphasic disability. *Canadian Journal of Neurological Sciences, 1,* 7–16.

Klich, R., Ireland, J., & Weidner, W. (1979). Articulatory and phonological aspects of consonant substitutions in apraxia of speech. *Cortex, 15,* 451–470.

Lane, V., & Samples, J. (1981). Facilitating communication skills in adult apraxics: Application of Blissymbols in a group setting. *Journal of Communication Disorders, 14,* 157–167.

LaPointe, L. (1969). *An investigation of isolated oral movements, oral sequencing motor abilities, and articulation of brain-injured adults.* Unpublished doctoral dissertation, University of Colorado.

LaPointe, L. (1977). Base-ten programmed stimulation: Task specifications, scoring and plotting performances in aphasia therapy. *Journal of Speech and Hearing Disorders, 42,* 90–105.

LaPointe, L. (1978). Aphasia therapy: Some principles and strategies for treatment. In D. Johns (Ed.), *Clinical management of neurogenic communicative disorders* (pp. 129–190). Boston: Little, Brown.

LaPointe, L. (1982). Neurogenic disorders of speech. In G. Shames & E. Wiig (Eds.), *Human communication disorders: An introduction* (pp. 370–400). Columbus, OH: Merrill.

LaPointe, L. (1983). Aphasia intervention with adults: Historical, present, and future approaches. In J. Miller, D. Yoder, & R. Schiefelbusch (Eds.), *Contemporary issues in language intervention* (Report No. 12, pp. 127–136). Rockville, MD: American Speech-Language-Hearing Association.

LaPointe, L. (1984). Sequential treatment of split lists: A case report. In J. Rosenbek, M. McNeil, & A. Aronson (Eds.), *Apraxia of speech: Physiology, acoustics, linguistics, management* (pp. 277–286). San Diego: College Hill Press.

LaPointe, L., & Horner, J. (1976). Repeated trials of words by patients with neurogenic phonological selection-sequencing impairment (apraxia of speech). In R. Brookshire (Ed.), *Clinical aphasiology: Conference proceedings* (pp. 261–277). Minneapolis: BRK Publishers.

LaPointe, L., & Horner, J. (1980). *Reading comprehension battery for aphasia*. Tygard, OR: C. C. Publications.

LaPointe, L., & Johns, D. (1975). Some phonemic characteristics in apraxia of speech. *Journal of Communication Disorders, 8*, 259–269.

LaPointe, L., & Wertz, R. (1974). Oral-movement abilities and articulatory characteristics of brain-injured adults. *Perceptual and Motor Skills, 39*, 39–46.

Lehman, H. (1967). Schizophrenia I.: Introduction and history. In A. Friedman & H. Kaplan (Eds.), *Textbook of psychiatry* (pp. 593–598). Baltimore: Williams & Wilkins.

Lesser, R. (1978). *Linguistic investigation of aphasia*. London: Edward Arnold.

Levin, H. (1981). Aphasia in closed head injury. In M. Sarno (Ed.), *Acquired aphasia* (pp. 427–463). New York: Academic Press.

Linebaugh, C. (1979). The dysarthrias of Shy-Drager syndrome. *Journal of Speech and Hearing Disorders, 44*, 55–60.

Linebaugh, C. (1984a). Mild aphasia. In A. Holland (Ed.), *Language disorders in adults* (pp. 113–131). San Diego: College Hill Press.

Linebaugh, C. (1984b). Treatment of flaccid dysarthria. In W. Perkins (Ed.), *Dysarthria and apraxia* (pp. 59–67). New York: Thieme-Stratton.

Linebaugh, C., Baird, J., Baird, C., & Armour, R. (1983). Special considerations for the development of microcomputer-based augmentative communication systems. In W. Berry (Ed.), *Clinical dysarthria* (pp. 295–303). San Diego: College Hill Press.

Linebaugh, C., & Wolfe, V. (1984). Relationships between articulation rate, intelligibility, and naturalness in spastic and ataxic speakers. In M. McNeil, J. Rosenbek, & A. Aronson (Eds.), *The dysarthrias: Physiology, acoustics, perception, management* (pp. 195–205). San Diego: College Hill Press.

Logemann, J., & Fisher, H. (1981). Vocal tract control in Parkinson's disease: Phonetic feature analysis of misarticulations. *Journal of Speech and Hearing Disorders, 46*, 348–352.

Logemann, J., Fisher, H., Boshes, B., & Blonsky, E. (1978). Frequency and cooccurrence of vocal tract dysfunctions in the speech of a large sample of Parkinson patients. *Journal of Speech and Hearing Disorders, 43*, 47–57.

Love, R., Hagerman, E., & Taimi, E. (1980). Speech performance, dysphagia, and oral reflexes in cerebral palsy. *Journal of Speech and Hearing Disorders, 45*, 59–75.

Lubinski, R. (1981). Environmental language intervention. In R. Chapey (Ed.), *Language intervention strategies in adult aphasia* (pp. 223–245). Baltimore: Williams & Wilkins.

Luchsinger, R., & Arnold, G. (1965). *Voice-speech-language: Clinical communicology – its physiology and pathology*. Belmont, CA: Wadsworth.

Ludlow, C. (1983). Identification and assessment of aphasic patients for language intervention. In J. Miller, D. Yoder, & R. Schiefelbusch (Eds.), *Contemporary issues in language intervention* (Report No. 12, pp. 75–81). Rockville, MD: American Speech-Language-Hearing Association.

Ludlow, C., & Bassich, C. (1983). The results of acoustic and perceptual assessment of two types of dysarthria. In W. Berry (Ed.), *Clinical dysarthria* (pp. 121–153). San Diego: College Hill Press.

Ludlow, C., & Bassich, C. (1984). Relationships between perceptual ratings and acoustic measures of hypokinetic speech. In M. McNeil, J. Rosenbek, & A. Aronson (Eds.), *The dysarthrias: Physiology, acoustics, perception, management* (pp. 163–195). San Diego: College Hill Press.

Marquardt, T., Reinhart, J., & Peterson, H. (1979). Markedness analysis of phonemic substitution errors in apraxia of speech. *Journal of Communication Disorders, 12,* 481–494.

Marquardt, T., & Sussman, H. (1984). The elusive lesion-apraxia of speech link in Broca's aphasia. In J. Rosenbek, M. McNeil, & A. Aronson (Eds.), *Apraxia of speech: Physiology, acoustics, linguistics, management* (pp. 91–112). San Diego: College Hill Press.

Marshall, R. (1981). Heightening auditory comprehension for aphasic patients. In R. Chapey (Ed.), *Language intervention strategies in adult aphasia* (pp. 297–328). Baltimore: Williams & Wilkins.

Marshall, R., & Phillips, D. (1983). Prognosis for improved verbal communication in aphasic stroke patients. *Archives of Physical Medicine and Rehabilitation, 64,* 597–600

Marshall, R., & Tompkins, C. (1981). Identifying behavior associated with verbal self-correction of aphasic clients. *Journal of Speech and Hearing Disorders, 46,* 168–173.

Martin, A., & Fedio, P. (1983). Word production and comprehension in Alzheimer's disease: The breakdown of semantic knowledge. *Brain and Language, 19,* 124–141.

Martin, A. D. (1978). *Therapy for dysarthria.* Paper presented at a conference on motor speech disorders. St. Vincent's Hospital, New York, NY.

Martin, A. D. (1981). An examination of Wepman's thought-centered therapy. In R. Chapey (Ed.), *Language intervention strategies in adult aphasia* (pp. 141–154). Baltimore: Williams & Wilkins.

Martin, A. D., & Rigrodsky, S. (1974). An investigation of phonological impairment in aphasia: Part I. *Cortex, 10,* 317–328.

Mayo Clinic. Section of neurology and section of physiology. (1964). *Clinical examinations in neurology.* Philadelphia: Saunders.

McDonald, E., & Schultz, A. (1973). Communication boards for cerebral palsied children. *Journal of Speech and Hearing Disorders, 38,* 73–88.

McNamara, R. (1983). A conceptual holistic approach to dysarthria treatment. In W. Berry (Ed.), *Clinical dysarthria* (pp. 191–201). San Diego: College Hill Press.

Mills, R., & Drummond, S. (1980, Nov.). *Analysis of impaired naming in language of confusion.* Paper presented at the meeting of the American Speech-Language-Hearing Association, Detroit.

Mohr, J. (1976). Broca's area and Broca's aphasia. In H. Whitaker & H. Whitaker (Eds.), *Studies in Neurolinguistics* (Vol. 1, pp. 201–235). New York: Academic Press.

Mohr, J. (1980). Revision of Broca aphasia and the syndrome of Broca's area infarction and its implications in aphasia therapy. In R. H. Brookshire (Ed.), *Clinical aphasiology conference proceedings* (pp. 1–16). Minneapolis: BRK.

Mohr, J., Pesin, M., Finkelstein, S., Funkenstein, H., Duncan, G., & Davis, K. (1978). Broca aphasia: Pathologic and clinical aspects. *Neurology, 28,* 311–324.

Muller-Suur, H. (1981). Spoerris' description of psychotic speech. In J. Darby (Ed.), *Speech evaluation in psychiatry* (pp. 349–357). New York: Grune & Stratton.

Muma, J., & McNeil, M. (1981). Intervention in aphasia: Psycho-socio-linguistic perspectives. In R. Chapey (Ed.), *Language intervention strategies in adult aphasia* (pp. 195–208). Baltimore: Williams & Wilkins.

Murry, T. (1983). The production of stress in three types of dysarthric speech. In W. Berry (Ed.), *Clinical dysarthria* (pp. 69–83). San Diego: College Hill Press.

Murry, T. (1984). Treatment for ataxic dysarthria. In W. Perkins (Ed.), *Dysarthria and apraxia* (pp. 75–89). New York: Thieme-Stratton.

Mysak, E., & Guarino, C. (1981). Self-adjusting therapy. In R. Chapey (Ed.), *Language intervention strategies in adult aphasia* (pp. 209–222). Baltimore: Williams & Wilkins.

Nemec, R., & Cohen, K. (1984). EMG feedback in the modification of hypertonia in spastic dysarthria: Case report. *Archives of Physical Medicine and Rehabilitation, 65*, 103–105.

Netsell, R. (1969). Changes in oropharyngeal cavity size of dysarthric children. *Journal of Speech and Hearing Research, 12*, 646–649.

Netsell, R. (1983). Speech-motor control: Theoretical issues with clinical impact. In W. Berry (Ed.), *Clinical dysarthria* (pp. 1–19). San Diego: College Hill Press.

Netsell, R. (1978). Physiologic recordings in the evaluation and rehabilitation of dysarthria. In L. Bradford (Ed.), *Communicative disorders: An audio journal for continuing education*. New York: Grune & Stratton.

Netsell, R. (1984). A neurobiologic view of the dysarthrias. In M. McNeil, J. Rosenbek, & A. Aronson (Eds.), *The dysarthrias: Physiology, acoustics, perception, management* (pp. 1–36). San Diego: College Hill Press.

Netsell, R., & Cleeland, C. (1973). Modification of lip hypotonia in dysarthria using EMG feedback. *Journal of Speech and Hearing Disorders, 38*, 131–139.

Netsell, R., & Daniel, B. (1979). Dysarthria in adults: Physiologic approach to rehabilitation. *Archives of Physical Medicine and Rehabilitation, 60*, 502–508.

Obler, L., & Albert, M. (1981). Language in the elderly aphasic and in the dementing patient. In M. Sarno (Ed.), *Acquired aphasia* (pp. 385–398). New York: Academic Press.

Obler, L., Albert, M., Estabrooks, N., & Nicholas, M. (1982, Oct.). *Noninformative speech in Alzheimer's dementia and in Wernicke's aphasia*. Paper presented at the meeting of the Academy of Aphasia, Lake Mohonk, NY.

O'Dwyer, N., Neilson, P., Guitar, B., Quinn, P., & Andrews, G. (1983). Control of upper airway structures during nonspeech tasks in normal and cerebral palsied subjects: EMG findings. *Journal of Speech and Hearing Research, 26*, 162–170.

Ostwald, P. (1981). Speech and schizophrenia. In J. Darby (Ed.), *Speech evaluation in psychiatry* (pp. 329–348). New York: Grune & Stratton.

Owens, R., & House, L. (1984). Decision-making processes in augmentative communication. *Journal of Speech and Hearing Disorders, 49*, 18–25.

Peacher, W. (1950). The etiology and differential diagnosis of dysarthria. *Journal of Speech and Hearing Disorders, 15*, 252–265.

Perkins, W. (Ed.). (1984). *Dysarthria and apraxia.* New York: Thieme-Stratton.

Platt, L., Andrews, G., & Howie, P. (1980a). Dysarthria of adult cerebral palsy: II. Phonemic analysis of articulation errors. *Journal of Speech and Hearing Research, 23,* 41–55.

Platt, L., Andrews, G., Young, M., & Quinn, P. (1980b). Dysarthria of adult cerebral palsy: I. Intelligibility and articulatory impairment. *Journal of Speech and Hearing Research, 23,* 28–40.

Porch, B. (1971). *Porch index of communicative ability II: Administration, scoring and interpretation* (rev. ed.). Palo Alto, CA: Consulting Psychologists Press.

Porch, B. (1981). Therapy subsequent to the PICA. In R. Chapey (Ed.), *Language intervention strategies in adult aphasia* (pp. 283–293). Baltimore: Williams & Wilkins.

Portnoy, R. (1979). Hyperkinetic dysarthria as an early indicator of impending tardive dyskinesia. *Journal of Speech and Hearing Disorders, 44,* 214–219.

Portnoy, R., & Aronson, A. (1982). Diadochokinetic syllable rate and regularity in normal and in spastic and ataxic dysarthric subjects. *Journal of Speech and Hearing Disorders, 47,* 324–328.

Powers, G., & Starr, C. (1974). The effects of muscle exercises on velopharyngeal gap and nasality. *Cleft Palate Journal, 11,* 28–35.

Putnam, A., & Hixon, T. (1984). Respiratory kinematics in speakers with motor neuron disease. In M. McNeil, J. Rosenbek, & A. Aronson (Eds.), *The dysarthrias: Physiology, acoustics, perception, management* (pp. 37–67). San Diego: College Hill Press.

Richman, J. (1968). Symbolic distortion in the vocabulary definitions of schizophrenia. In H. Vetter (Ed.), *Language behavior in schizophrenia* (pp. 49–57). Springfield, IL: Thomas.

Riedel, K. (1981). Auditory comprehension in aphasia. In M. Sarno (Ed.), *Acquired aphasia* (pp. 215–269). New York: Academic Press.

Rochester, S. (1980). Thought disorders and language use in schizophrenia. In R. Rieber (Ed.), *Applied psycholinguistics and mental health* (pp. 11–67). New York: Plenum Press.

Rochester, S., & Martin, J. (1979). *Crazy talk: A study of the discourse of schizophrenic speakers.* New York: Plenum Press.

Rollin, W. (1984). Family therapy and the aphasic adult. In J. Eisenson, *Adult aphasia* (pp. 252–282). Englewood Cliffs, NJ: Prentice-Hall.

Rosenbek, J. (1978). Treating apraxia of speech. In D. Johns (Ed.), *Clinical management of neurogenic communicative disorders* (pp. 191–241). Boston: Little, Brown.

Rosenbek, J. (1983). Some challenges for clinical aphasiologists. In J. Miller, D. Yoder, & R. Schiefelsbusch (Ed.), *Contemporary issues in language intervention* (Report No. 12, pp. 317–325). Rockville, MD: American Speech-Language-Hearing Association.

Rosenbek, J. (1984). Treatment for apraxia of speech in adults. In W. Perkins (Ed.), *Dysarthria and apraxia* (pp. 49–56). New York: Thieme-Stratton.

Rosenbek, J., Hansen, R., Baughman, C., & Lemme, M. (1974). Treatment of developmental apraxia of speech: A case study. *Language, Speech, and Hearing Services in the Schools, 5*, 13–22.

Rosenbek, J., Kent, R., & LaPointe, L. (1984). Apraxia of speech: An overview and some perspectives. In J. Rosenbek, M. McNeil, & A. Aronson (Eds.), *Apraxia of speech: Physiology, acoustics, linguistics, management* (pp. 1–72). San Diego: College Hill Press.

Rosenbek, J., & LaPointe, L. (1978). The dysarthrias: Description, diagnosis, and treatment. In D. Johns (Ed.), *Clinical management of neurogenic communicative disorders* (pp. 251–310). Boston: Little, Brown.

Rosenbek, J., & LaPointe, L. (1982). A physiological approach to the dysarthrias. *Journal of Speech and Hearing Disorders, 47*, 334.

Rosenbek, J., Lemme, M., Ahern, M., Harris, E., & Wertz; R. (1973). A treatment for apraxia of speech in adults. *Journal of Speech and Hearing Disorders, 38*, 462–472.

Rosenbek, J., Wertz, R., & Darley, F. (1973). Oral sensation and perception in apraxia of speech. *Journal of Speech and Hearing Research, 16*, 22–36.

Rubow, R. (1984). Role of feedback, reinforcement, and compliance in training and transfer in biofeedback-based rehabilitation of motor speech disorders. In M. McNeil, J. Rosenbek, & A. Aronson (Eds.), *The dysarthrias: Physiology, acoustics, perception, management* (pp. 207–230). San Diego: College Hill Press.

Rubow, R., Rosenbek, J., Collins, M., & Celesia, G. (1984). Reduction of hemifacial spasm and dysarthria following EMG biofeedback. *Journal of Speech and Hearing Disorders, 49*, 26–33.

Rubow, R., Rosenbek, J., Collins, M., & Longstreth, D. (1982). Vibro-tactile stimulation for intersystemic reorganization in the treatment of apraxia of speech. *Archives of Physical Medicine and Rehabilitation, 63*, 150–153.

Rumke, H., & Nijdam, S. (1958). Aphasia and delusion. *Folia Psychiatric Neurologic Neurochir. Nerl., 61*, 623–629.

Salzinger, K., Portnoy, S., Feldman, R., & Patenaud-Lane, J. (1980). From method to madness: The Close procedure in the study of psychopathology. In R. Rieber (Ed.), *Applied psycholinguistics and mental health* (pp. 93–113). New York: Plenum Press.

Sands, E., Freeman, F., & Harris, K. (1978). Progressive changes in articulatory patterns in verbal apraxia: A longitudinal case study. *Brain and Language, 6*, 97–105.

Sarno, J. (1981). Emotional aspects of aphasia. In M. Sarno (Ed.), *Acquired aphasia* (pp. 465–484). New York: Academic Press.

Sarno, M. (1969). *Functional communication profile*. New York: Institute of Rehabilitative Medicine.

Sarno, M. (1980). The nature of verbal impairment after closed head injury. *Journal of Nervous and Mental Disease, 168*, 685–692.

Sarno, M. (1981). Recovery and rehabilitation in aphasia. In M. Sarno (Ed.), *Acquired aphasia* (pp. 485–529). New York: Academic Press.

Schuell, H. (1957). A short examination for aphasia. *Neurology, 7*, 625–634.

Schuell, H. (1972). *The Minnesota test for differential diagnosis of aphasia*. Minneapolis: Univ. of Minn. Press.

Schuell, H., Jenkins, J., & Jimenez-Pabon, E. (1964). *Aphasia in adults: Diagnosis, prognosis, and treatment*. New York: Hoeber Medical Division, Harper.

Schwartz, M. (1984). What the classical aphasia categories can't do for us and why. *Brain and Language, 21*, 3–8.

Seron, X., DeLoche, G., Moulard, G., & Rouselle, M. (1980). A computer-based therapy for the treatment of aphasic subjects with writing disorders. *Journal of Speech and Hearing Disorders, 45*, 45–58.

Shane, H., & Bashir, A. (1980). Election criteria for the adoption of an augmentative communication system: Preliminary considerations. *Journal of Speech and Hearing Disorders, 45*, 408–414.

Shane, H., & Darley, F. (1978). The effect of auditory rhythmic stimulation on articulatory accuracy in apraxia of speech. *Cortex, 14*, 444–450.

Shankweiler, D., & Harris, K. (1966). An experimental approach to the problem of articulation in aphasia. *Cortex, 2*, 277–292.

Shapiro, T. (1979). *Clinical psycholinguistics*. New York: Plenum Press.

Shaughnessy, A., Netsell, R., & Farrage, J. (1983). Treatment for a four-year-old with a palatal lift prosthesis. In W. Berry (Ed.), *Clinical dysarthria* (pp. 217–230). San Diego: College Hill Press.

Shelton, R., Hahn, E., & Morris, H. (1968). Diagnosis and therapy. In D. Spriestersbach & D. Sherman (Eds.), *Cleft palate and communication* (pp. 225–268). New York: Academic Press.

Shewan, C. (1980). *Auditory comprehension test for sentences*. Chicago: Biolinguistics Clinical Institute.

Shewan, C., Leeper, H., & Booth, J. (1984). An analysis of voice onset time (VOT) in aphasic and normal subjects. In J. Rosenbek, M. McNeil, & A. Aronson (Eds.), *Apraxia of speech: Physiology, acoustics, linguistics, management* (pp. 197–220). San Diego: College Hill Press.

Silverman, F. (1984). Dysarthria: Communication-augmentative systems for adults without speech. In W. Perkins (Ed.), *Dysarthria and apraxia* (pp. 115–121). New York: Thieme-Stratton.

Simmons, N. (1983). Acoustic analysis of ataxic dysarthria: An approach to monitoring treatment. In W. Berry (Ed.), *Clinical dysarthria* (pp. 283–294). San Diego: College Hill Press.

Sklar, M. (1966). *Sklar aphasia scale*. Los Angeles: Western Psychological Services.

Sparks, R. (1981). Melodic intonation therapy. In R. Chapey (Ed.), *Language intervention strategies in adult aphasia* (pp. 265–282). Baltimore: Williams & Wilkins.

Sparks, R., & Holland, A. (1976). Method: Melodic intonation therapy for aphasia. *Journal of Speech and Hearing Disorders, 41*, 287–297.

Spreen, O., & Benton, A. (1969). *Neurosensory center comprehensive examination for aphasia*. Victoria, B.C., Canada: Univ. of Victoria Neuropsychology Laboratory.

Spreen, O., & Risser, A. (1981). Assessment of aphasia. In M. Sarno (Ed.), *Acquired aphasia* (pp. 67–127). New York: Academic Press.

Square, P. (1981). *Auditory perceptual abilities of patients with apraxia of speech.* Unpublished doctoral dissertation, Kent State University.

Steadman, J., Ferris, C., & Rhodine, N. (1980). Prosthetic communication device. *Archives of Physical Medicine and Rehabilitation, 61*, 93–97.

Stein, S. (1981). Medical management of cerebrovascular accidents. In R. Chapey (Ed.), *Language intervention strategies in adult aphasia* (pp. 15–29). Baltimore: Williams & Wilkins.

Stengel, E. (1964). Speech disorders and mental disorders. In A. DeReuck & M. O'Connor (Eds.), *Disorders of language* (pp. 285–292). London: Churchill.

Taylor, M. (1964). Language therapy. In G. Burr (Ed.), *The aphasic adult: Evaluation and rehabilitation* (pp. 130–160). Charlottesville, VA: Wayside Press.

Tikofsky, R. (1984). Assessment of aphasic disorders. In J. Eisenson (Ed.), *Adult aphasia* (pp. 117–149). Englewood Cliffs, NJ: Prentice-Hall.

Tikofsky, R., & Tikosfsky, R. (1964). Intelligibility measures of dysarthric speech. *Journal of Speech and Hearing Research, 7,* 325–333.

Tompkins, C., Marshall, R., & Phillips, D. (1980). Aphasic patients in a rehabilitation program: Scheduling speech and language services. *Archives of Physical Medicine and Rehabilitation, 66*, 252–257.

Trost, J., & Canter, G. (1974). Apraxia of speech in patients with Brocha's aphasia: A study of phonemic production accuracy and error patterns. *Brain and Language, 1*, 63–79.

Trost, J., & Canter, G. (1974). Apraxia of speech in patients with Broca's aphasia: A study of phonemic production accuracy and error patterns. *Brain and Language, 1*, 63–79.

Vignolo, L. (1964). Evaluation of aphasia and language rehabilitation: A retrospective exploratory study. *Cortex, 1*, 344–367.

Warren, R. (1977). Rehearsal for naming in apraxia of speech. In R. Brookshire (Ed.), *Clinical aphasiology: Conference proceedings* (pp. 80–90). Minneapolis: BRK Publishers.

Weinstein, E. (1956). Changes in language pattern as adaptive mechanisms. *Proceedings of the American Psychopathic Association, 46*, 262–271.

Weinstein, E., Lyerly, O., Cole, M., & Ozer, M. (1966). Meaning in jargon aphasia. *Cortex, 2*, 165–187.

Weismer, G. (1984). Articulatory characteristics of Parkinsonian dysarthria: Segmental and phrase-level timing, spirantization, and glottal-supraglottal coordination. In M. McNeil, J. Rosenbek, & A. Aronson (Eds.), *The dysarthrias: Physiology, acoustics, perception, management* (pp. 101–130). San Diego: College Hill Press.

Wepman, J. (1951). *Recovery from aphasia*. New York: Ronald Press.

Wepman, J. (1953). A conceptual model for the processes involved in recovery from aphasia. *Journal of Speech and Hearing Disorders, 18*, 4–13.

Wepman, J., & Jones, L. (1961). *The language modalities test for aphasia.* Chicago: Education Industry Service.

Wertz, R. (1978). Neuropathologies of speech and language: An introduction to patient management. In D. F. Johns (Ed.), *Clinical management of neurogenic communicative disorders* (pp. 1–101). Boston: Little, Brown.

Wertz, R. (1981). Aphasia management: The speech pathologist's role. *Seminars in Speech, Language and Hearing, 4*, 315–331.

Wertz, R. (1982). *Language deficit in aphasia and dementia: The same as, different from, or both*. Paper presented at the meeting of the Clinical Aphasiology Conference, Oshkosh, WI.

Wertz, R. (1983a). Language intervention context and setting for the aphasic adult: When? In J. Miller, D. Yoder, & R. Schiefelbusch (Eds.), *Contemporary issues in language intervention* (Report No. 12, pp. 196–220). Rockville, MD: American Speech-Language-Hearing Association.

Wertz, R. (1983b). A philosophy of aphasia therapy: Some things that patients do not say but you can see if you listen. *Communicative Disorders, 8*, 1–17.

Wertz, R. (1984a). Language disorders in adults: State of the clinical art. In A. Holland (Ed.), *Language disorders in adults* (pp. 1–77). San Diego: College Hill Press.

Wertz, R. (1984b). Response to treatment in patients with apraxia of speech. In J. Rosenbek, M. McNeil, & A. Aronson (Eds.), *Apraxia of speech: Physiology, acoustics, linguistics, management* (pp. 257–276). San Diego: College Hill Press.

Wertz, R., Collins, M., Weiss, D., Kurtzke, J., Friden, T., Brookshire, R., Pierce, J., Holtzapple, P., Hubbard, D., Porch, B., West, J., Davis, L., Matovitch, V., Morley, G., & Resurreccion, E. (1981). Veterans Administration cooperative study in aphasia: A comparison of individual and group treatment. *Journal of Speech and Hearing Research, 24*, 580–594.

Wertz, R., LaPointe, L., & Rosenbek, J. (1984). *Apraxia of speech in adults*. New York: Grune & Stratton.

Whitehorn, J., & Zipf, G. (1943). Schizophrenic language. *Archives of Neurologic Psychiatry, 49*, 831–851.

Wilson, R., & Antablin, J. (1980). A picture identification task as an estimate of the word-recognition performance of non-verbal adults. *Journal of Speech and Hearing Disorders, 45*, 223–237.

Wilson, R., Kaszniak, A., Bacon, L., Fox, J., & Kelly, M. (1982). Facial recognition memory in dementia. *Cortex, 18*, 329–336.

Wilson, R., Kaszniak, A., & Fox, J. (1981). Remote memory in senile dementia. *Cortex, 17*, 41–48.

Wolfe, V., Ratusknik, D., & Penn, R. (1981). Long-term effects on speech of chronic cerebellar stimulation in cerebral palsy. *Journal of Speech and Hearing Disorders, 46*, 286–290.

Wykes, T., & Leff, J. (1982). Disordered speech: Differences between manics and schizophrenics. *Brain and Language, 15*, 117–124.

Wynne, R. (1963). The influence of hospitalization on the verbal behavior of chronic schizophrenics. *British Journal of Psychiatry, 109*, 380–389.

Yoder, D., & Kraat, A. (1983). Intervention issues in nonspeech communication. In J. Miller, D. Yoder, & R. Schiefelbusch (Eds.), *Contemporary issues in language intervention* (Report No. 12, pp. 27–51). Rockville, MD: American Speech-Language-Hearing Association.

Yorkston, K., & Beukelman, D. (1980). A clinician-judged technique for quantifying dysarthric speech based on single-word intelligibility. *Journal of Communication Disorders, 13*, 15–31.

Yorkston, K., & Beukelman, D. (1981a). Communication efficiency of dysarthric speakers as measured by sentence intelligibility and speaking rate. *Journal of Speech and Hearing Disorders, 46*, 296–301.

Yorkston, K., & Beukelman, D. (1981b). *Assessment of intelligibility of dysarthric speech.* Tigard, OR: C. C. Publications.

Yorkston, K., & Beukelman, D. (1981c). Ataxic dysarthria: Treatment sequences based on intelligibility and prosodic considerations. *Journal of Speech and Hearing Disorders, 46*, 398–404.

Yorkston, K., & Beukelman, D. (1983). The influence of judge familiarization with the speaker on dysarthric speech intelligibility. In W. Berry (Ed.), *Clinical dysarthria* (pp. 153–163). San Diego: College Hill Press.

Yorkston, K., Beukelman, D., Minifie, F., & Sapir, S. (1984). Assessment of stress patterning. In M. McNeil, J. Rosenbek, & A. Aronson (Eds.), *The dysarthrias: Physiology, acoustics, perception, management* (pp. 131–162). San Diego: College Hill Press.

Yorkston, K., & Dowden, P. (1984). Nonspeech language and communication systems. In A. Holland (Ed.), *Language disorders in adults* (pp. 283–312). San Diego: College Hill Press.

Yoss, K., & Darley, F. (1974). Therapy in developmental apraxia of speech. *Language, Speech, and Hearing Services in the Schools, 5*, 23–31.

Zangwill, O. (1964). Intelligence in aphasia. In A. DeReuck & M. O'Connor (Eds.), *Disorders of language* (pp. 261–274). London: Churchill.

Harvey Halpern is a Professor in the Department of Communication Arts and Sciences at Queens College as well as on the doctoral faculty in speech and hearing sciences at the City University of New York. He has published numerous articles, several chapters, and was editor of the Bobbs-Merrill series Studies in Communicative Disorders, to which he contributed *Adult Aphasia*; he is currently editor of the series Pro-Ed Studies in Communicative Disorders. He has delivered over 65 professional papers, including a number of short courses, and has contributed recorded material to several tape libraries. He was a postdoctoral fellow at the Mayo Clinic and is a member of the Academy of Aphasia. He is a member with licensure in speech pathology and a past president of the New York State Speech-Language-Hearing Association. He is also a member with certification in speech pathology, a former Legislative Councilor, and a Fellow of the American Speech-Language-Hearing Association.